CELEBRATIONS

LIVING LIFE TO THE FULLEST

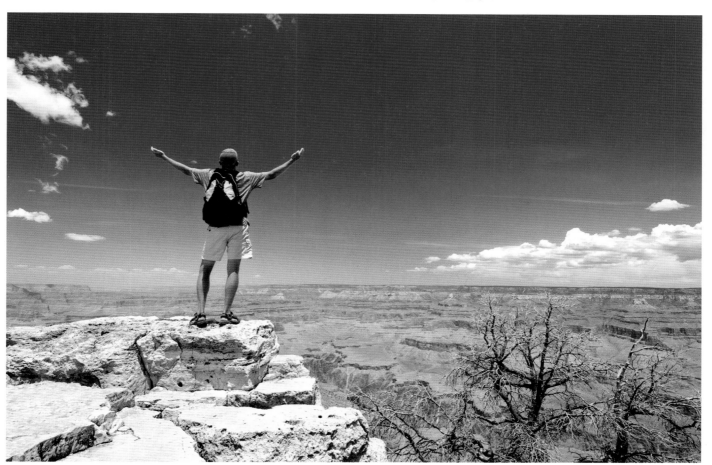

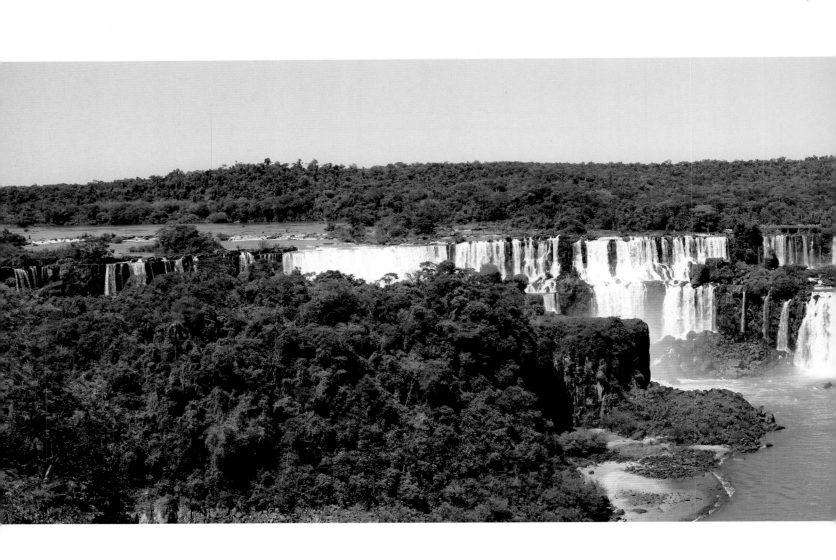

CELEBRATIONS

General Conference of Seventh-day Adventists Health Ministries Department

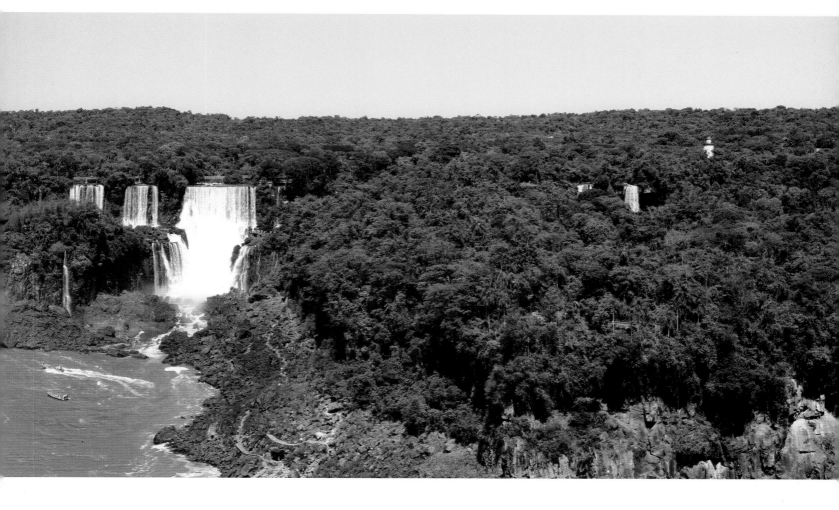

Editor: Sandra Blackmer
Editorial Assistant: Elizabeth Pettit
Proofreaders: Gary Swanson, Erica Richards, Stephen Chavez
Cover Designer: Merle Poirier
Interior Designer: Merle Poirier

ISBN 978-1-4652-0940-5   Hardbound Edition
ISBN 978-1-4652-0941-2   Softcover Edition

Printed in the United States of America
10 9 8 7 6 5 4 3 2 1

We dedicate this book to you, the reader, who we
hope will find within its pages something to
help you to celebrate living.

_____

"When text, images, and design work wonderfully together, readers everywhere rejoice. When they powerfully communicate the principles and practices of a healthful lifestyle, there is cause for *CELEBRATIONS*—a volume that will add abundance to your life and life to your years. The message of this remarkable book is both simple and profound: You can live the better, happier life that you've always dreamed of.

—*Bill Knott, executive publisher and editor,* Adventist Review *and* Adventist World

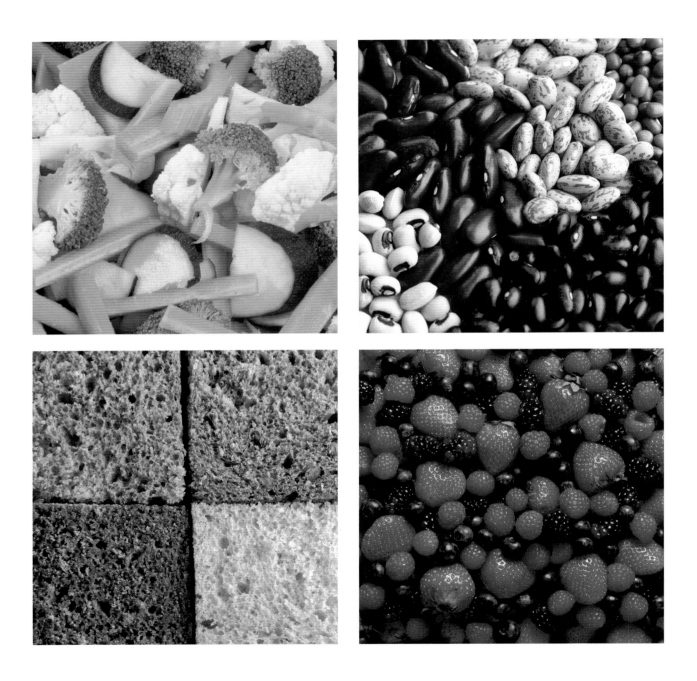

ACKNOWLEDGMENTS

It's with deep appreciation that we acknowledge and thank those who contributed to the development of this book:

- *Soli Deo Gloria* — To God be the glory.
- The gracious donor, Judy Thomas, who supplied the funds to produce *CELEBRATIONS*.
- Stoy Proctor, for his meticulous help with research.
- Elizabeth Pettit, who spent countless hours typing chapters, researching information, assisting the editor with various tasks, assisting the designer by securing photos, and a myriad of other duties too numerous to mention.
- Laura Sanchez, Nancy Thomas, and Iris Shull, for their fastidious assistance.
- Sandra Blackmer, who served as project manager and editor.
- Merle Poirier, who designed the book.
- Gary Swanson, Erica Richards, and Steve Chavez, who proofread the material.
- Rosalind Landless, who authored the Life-Application Questions.

We are profoundly grateful to these individuals, without whom the production and printing of this book would not have been possible.

Allan Handysides, Peter Landless,
Kathleen Kuntaraf, and Fred Hardinge

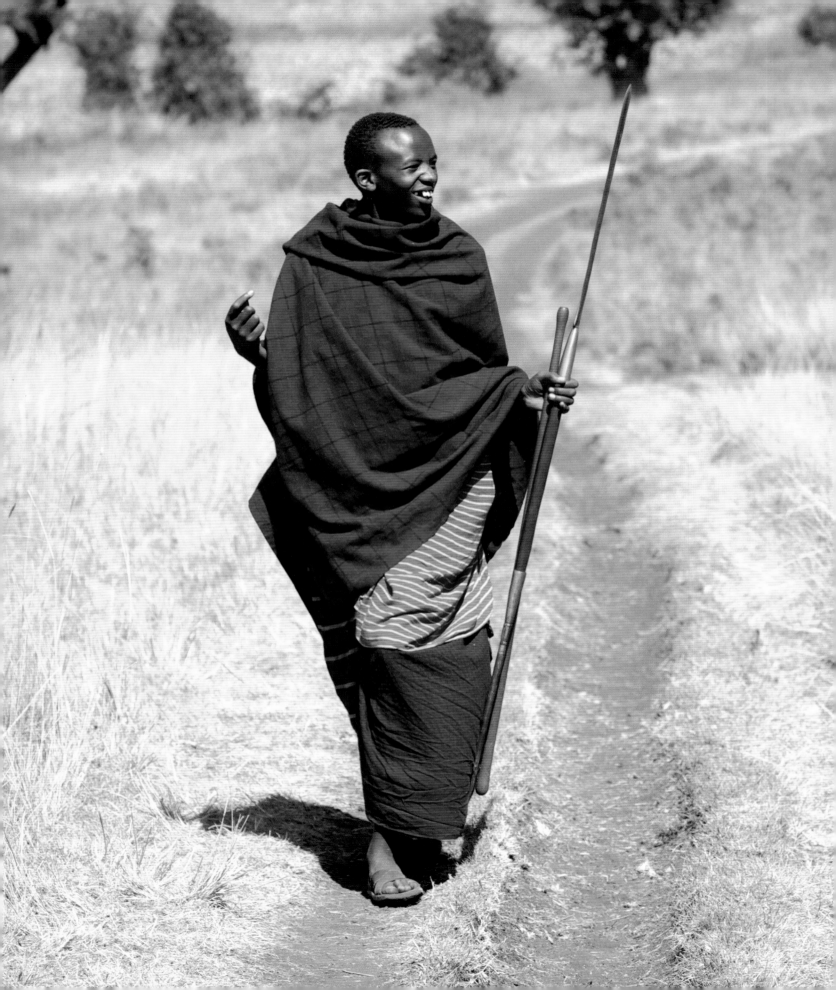

"*CELEBRATIONS* places the healthful-living focus right where it should be: on God's desire for His people to be happy, healthy, and energized for joyful mission and outreach service to others. Biblical principles and evidenced-based studies provide the foundation for these "secrets" to acquiring good health; yet the doctors present them in a way that makes healthful-lifestyle practices attainable for all. Once you begin leafing through the pages, the stunning photography arrests your imagination and won't let you put the book down. This is beneficial reading material for everyone as we carry out the principles of the medical missionary work of Jesus Christ, who is the Master Physician and soon-coming Savior.

—Ted N. C. Wilson, president, General Conference of Seventh-day Adventists

EACH PAGE of this beautifully produced book reflects a balanced, wholistic approach to good health that's firmly grounded in spiritual values. In *CELEBRATIONS*, the Health Ministries Department of the General Conference has produced an evidence-backed, step-by-step guide to a lifestyle that embraces not just physical well-being but also the ability to live fully, breathe freely, and experience a sense of joy and peace. I pray that readers will be inspired by its straightforward, easy-to-follow presentation, and that they will come to know what it truly means to live a "more abundant life."

—Jan Paulsen, former president (1999-2010), General Conference of Seventh-day Adventists

TOTAL HEALTH—spiritual, mental, and physical—is something to be celebrated. The book *CELEBRATIONS* embraces all three, and encourages us to live life to the full. I wholeheartedly endorse and appreciate the publication of this book. I know from my own personal experience the blessings of exercising body, mind, and spirit. My prayer is that the reader will have this experience too.

—Delbert Baker, a general vice president, General Conference, and advisor to the Health Ministries Department

A MOST APPEALING and helpful book. The authors have valued balance in a wide-ranging approach to living. Their recommendations are guided by common sense, a deep understanding of human physiology, and scientific results regarding lifestyle and health when these are available.

—Gary Fraser, M.B., Ch.B., Ph.D., MPH, professor of medicine and epidemiology, and director of Adventist Health Study-2, Loma Linda University

THIS IS AN ATTRACTIVE, aesthetically pleasing presentation of common sense lifestyle habits and practices that most adults and even youngsters should adopt for a healthier life—preventive medicine in action. It promotes lifestyle as primary health care, an intervention so much needed amid the current pandemic of obesity and diabetes (diabesity), affecting so many parts of the world. Numerous references to peer-reviewed scientific literature promote its health recommendations as plausible and evidence-based. This book turns the pedestrian, needed, and sometimes onerous health-habit changes into beneficial and sustainable celebrations!

—E. Albert Reece, M.D., Ph.D., MBA, vice president for Medical Affairs, University of Maryland John Z. and Akiko K. Bowers Distinguished Professor and dean, University of Maryland School of Medicine

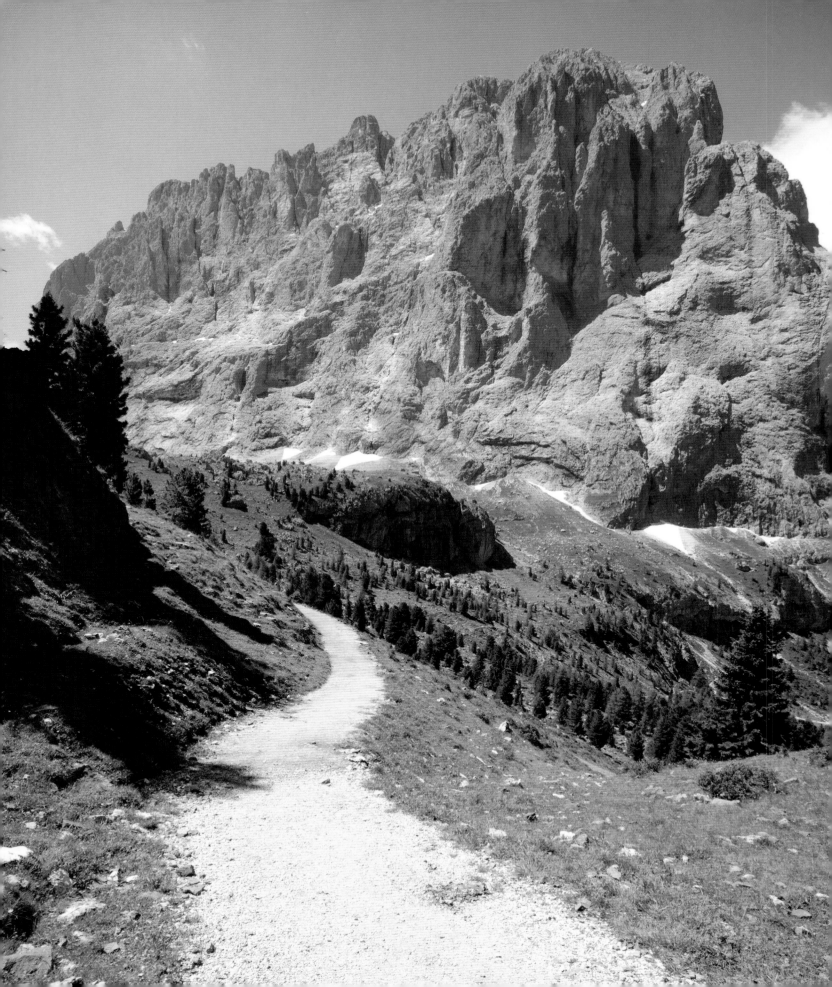

CONTENTS

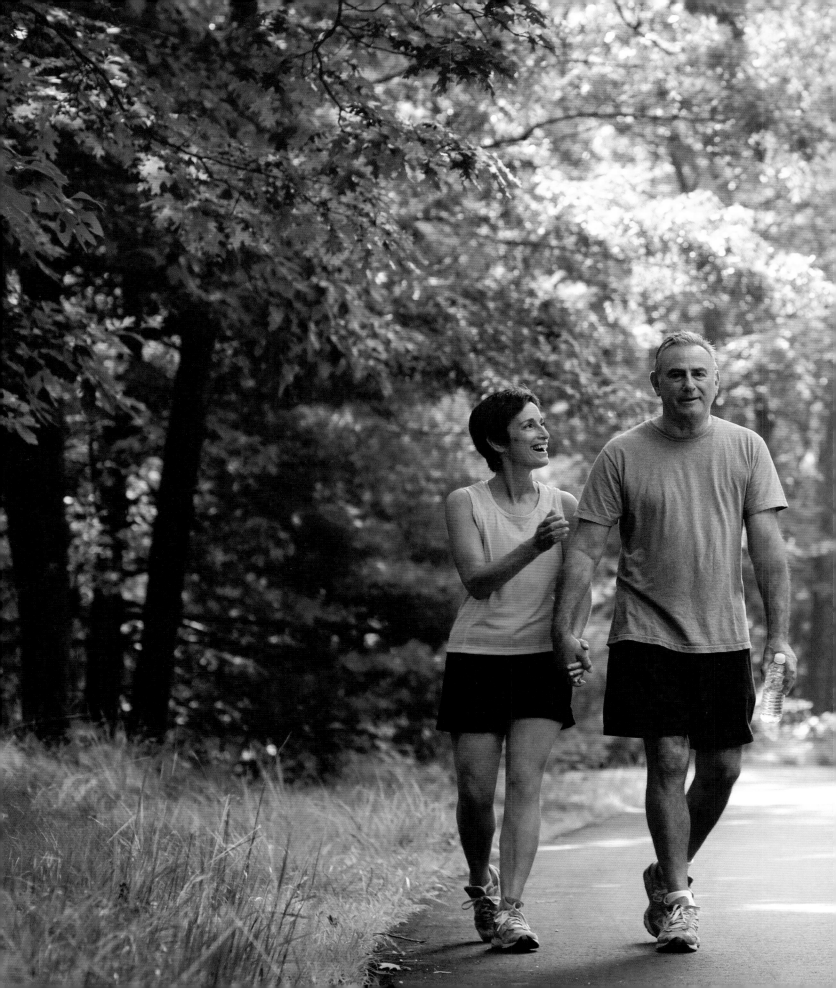

INTRODUCTION

Data collected in several studies on Seventh-day Adventists have shown conclusively that, on average, those who follow the whole-health principles outlined in this CELEBRATIONS® program live some 10 years longer than comparable Adventists who do not follow the principles—and of the general public who collectively live the "American lifestyle" of consuming a high-fat, high-sugar, refined-food diet and not exercising regularly.

This book will present you with a number of challenging concepts and significant choices. These choices cover a diverse selection of lifestyle options, such as the mental, emotional, physical, spiritual, and social aspects of life.

CELEBRATIONS® is an acronym for 12 healthful living principles: (1) choices, (2) exercise, (3) liquid, (4) environment, (5) belief, (6) rest, (7) air, (8) temperance, (9) integrity, (10) optimism, (11) nutrition, and (12) social support and service.

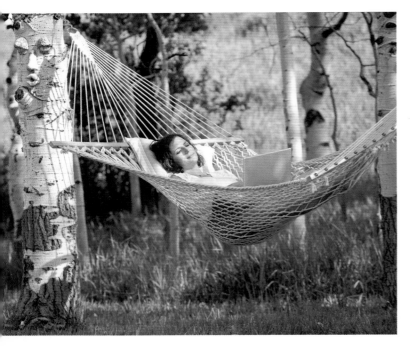

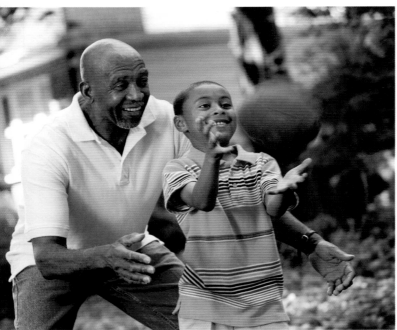

We also make four promises to our readers:

1. The choices are yours to make, and we honor your individual rights and responsibility.

2. We as Seventh-day Adventists believe in a Creator God and will speak openly and sensitively of this belief. As a group, we are some of the world's strongest believers in religious freedom, and we will not seek to coerce but to show the joy of embracing a healthful lifestyle.

3. We will seek at all times to present scientifically supported material that will enhance the quality of your life.

4. We are interested in you as individuals—your prosperity and health—and CELEBRATIONS® was not developed for profit. This is a nonprofit venture.

Choosing health and celebrating the joy of life should be an intentional decision that is well-informed and freely made. As early twentieth-century politician William Jennings Bryan said, "Destiny is no matter of chance. It is a matter of choice. It is not a thing to be waited for; it is a thing to be achieved."

This entire philosophy of CELEBRATIONS® involves individuals making their own choices backed by evidence-based information—a condensation of what has been called the "Adventist lifestyle."

Central to the Adventist philosophy on health is an interest in every aspect of human life, or wholesome living. The "whole" here relates to body, mind, emotions, spiritual dimensions, and social interactions.

It is, therefore, with pleasure that we bring you this offering of an acronym that carries within it both the secrets of a healthful lifestyle and an exuberant appreciation of the joy of living well.

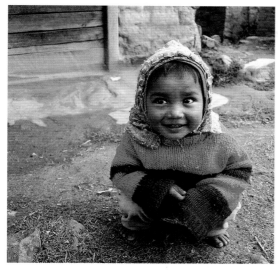

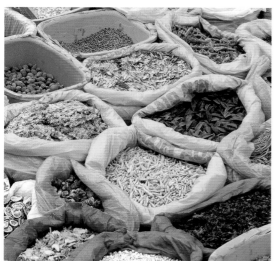

CONTRIBUTORS

Chapter Authors

Allan R. Handysides, M.B., Ch.B., FRCPC, FRCSC, FACOG

Director, Health Ministries Department,
General Conference of Seventh-day Adventists

Fred G. Hardinge, DrPh, RD, FADA

Associate Director for Nutrition, Health Ministries Department,
General Conference of Seventh-day Adventists

Kathleen Kiem Hoa Oey Kuntaraf, M.D., MPH

Associate Director for Prevention, Health Ministries Department,
General Conference of Seventh-day Adventists

Peter N. Landless, M.B., B.Ch., M.Med., MFGP (SA), FCP (SA), FACC, FASNC

Associate Director, Health Ministries Department, General Conference of
Seventh-day Adventists, and Executive Director, International Commission
for the Prevention of Alcoholism and Drug Dependency (ICPA)

Researcher

Stoy Proctor, M.Div., MPH

Associate Director for Nutrition and Smoking Cessation, Health Ministries
Department, General Conference of Seventh-day Adventists, and a researcher
for this book.

Life-Applications Author

Rosalind Landless

Database and Web specialist, International Personnel Resources and Services,
General Conference of Seventh-day Adventists

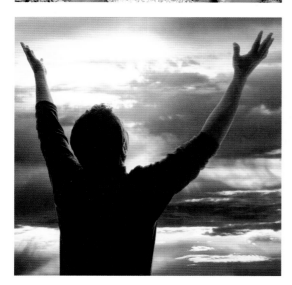

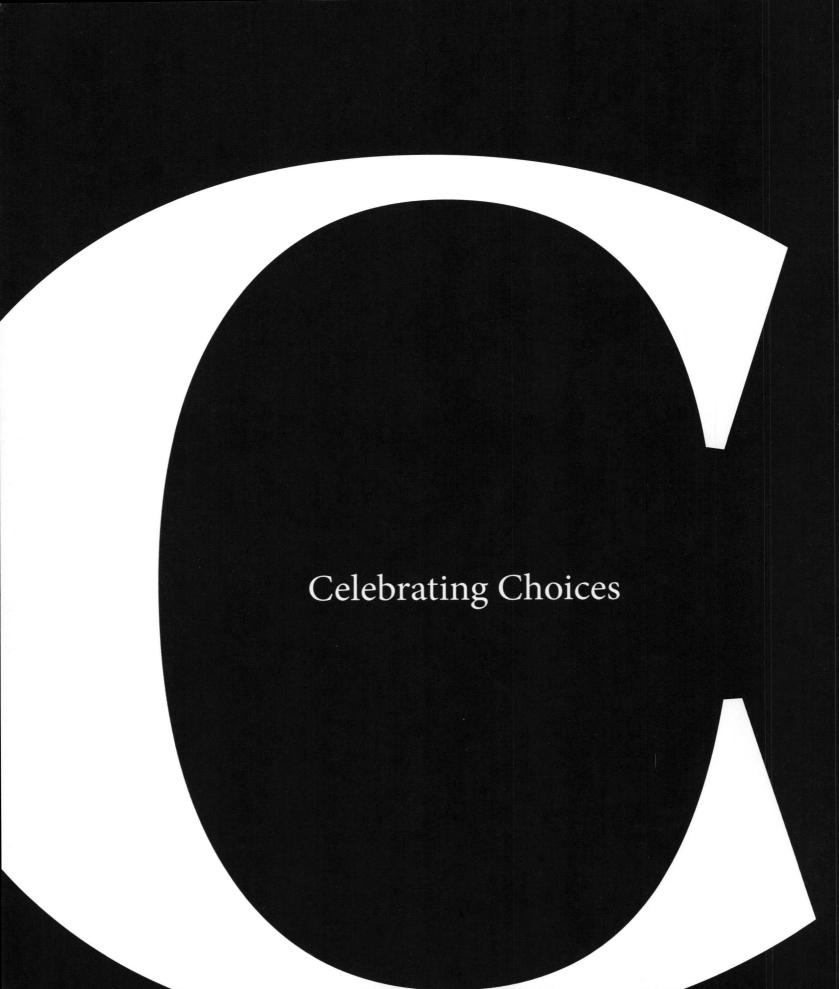

Celebrating Choices

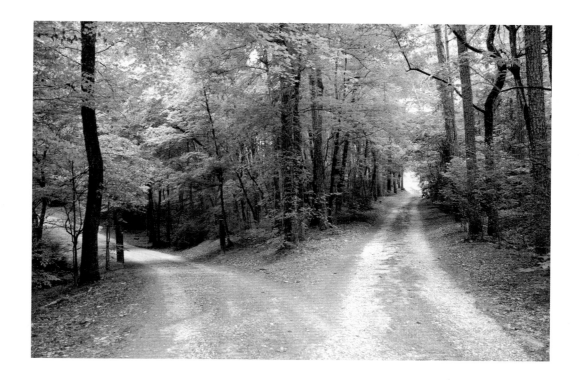

Some 100 years ago two team leaders adopted the same goal: they both sought to be the first to lead an expedition to the South Pole.

Once made, the decision presented them with countless choices: selecting the clothing to wear, the food to eat, and, most important, the mode of transport.

Roald Amundsen, the Norwegian explorer, gleaned from Inuit methodology the best type of equipment and clothing to use. He chose dogs to pull the sleds. He placed his supplies and food-

stuffs strategically along the early part of the proposed route to travel before the main expedition set off, thereby lessening the loads his dogs would have to pull. He carefully considered every detail, and from his informed base he made decisions as to how to proceed.

Robert Falcon Scott, however, a British naval officer, chose to use ponies and "modern" motorized sledges. He was a brave and daring man, but apparently did not pay the same attention to Inuit methodology as did Amundsen. His motorized sleds ceased function-

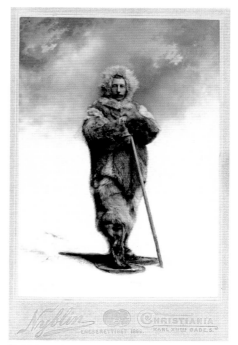

Roald Amundsen

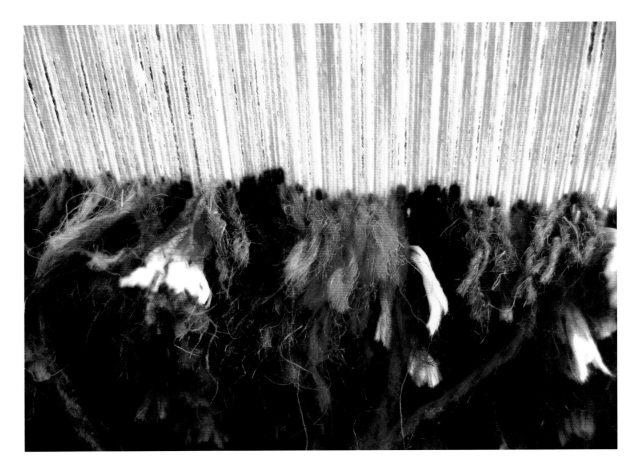

ing after a few days, and the ponies could not stand the frigid conditions. By the time he and his team reached the Transantarctic Mountains, the ponies were in such poor condition they had to be killed. Scott arrived at the South Pole to find that Amundsen had beaten him to the goal.

The outcome for one team was triumph; for the other, death and disaster. The diaries of Scott's heroic team chronicled a story of frostbite, starvation, and eventually death on the return journey from the pole.

Decisions made or neglected by Amundsen and Scott represented choices. Some were made very consciously and intentionally; others were possibly influenced by emotion, personality, culture, or whim. Brave and courageous though Scott and his men were, they suffered the consequences of their choices and decisions, perhaps made in ignorance, but nevertheless lethal in outcome.[1]

CHOICES—THE CRADLE OF DESTINY

Choices often determine our destiny. To a large extent even our health can be determined by the choices we make on how we live, the risks we take, and the balance we seek in life. We each come into the world with an endowment for health that may vary from that of others, but how we care for the gift of our health influences the expression of our genetic capacities.

The intricacies of handmade Asian rugs are remarkable and often represent hundreds of thousands and sometimes even millions of individual choices. For those rugs with 800 hand-tied knots per square inch, the maker has to select a colored thread to create the pattern 800 times. In the overall pattern, the subtle variety in the shapes making up the whole speaks to the individuality of each knot.

Our lives are patterned in a similar way. Every day we make countless seemingly insignificant decisions, the sum of which determines the overall fabric of our lives.

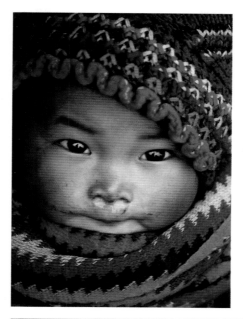

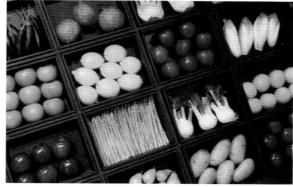

INTENTIONALITY IS KEY

Intentionality in decision-making brings direction and order to our lives. Successful people generally set goals and objectives; highly successful individuals make evidence-based decisions that move them deliberately toward those goals.

Unfortunately, some decisions made in youth—as a result of ignorance, rebellion, or stubbornness—can have lifelong repercussions. Similarly, poor parenting practices can encumber children with a lifetime of consequences. In many cases the current epidemic

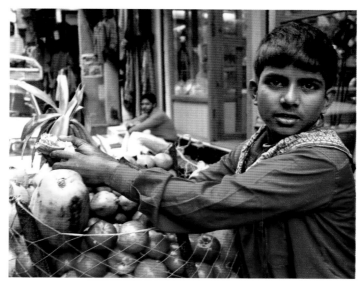

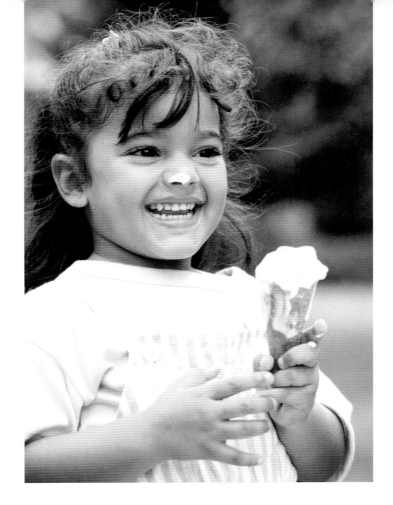

of obesity in children in the Western world reflects parental resignation to allowing too much electronic entertainment at the expense of physical activity. Fast and convenient foods replace simple, unrefined, natural foods. The immediate gratification of fast, oily, and high-calorie foods pleases both parents and children, but the consequences of such choices may last a lifetime. Once formed, fat cells persist for years, awaiting excess calories to be stored as fat. Chubby children are obese adults-in-waiting. The fat baby carries a legacy for life that perhaps reflects the parental inability or unwillingness to control caloric intake. Conscious intentionality is an important part of making such choices.

CHOICE AND FREEDOM

Choice and freedom are closely linked. Many correctional services seek to discipline by limiting available choices. In most societies even the greatest of freedoms permits only the choices that do not negatively impact others, because freedom to choose does not permit the freedom to harm others and escape consequences.

We have "free will" to choose, provided previous choices have not enslaved or—as it were—imprisoned us. Choices, however, are not always easy to make, yet avoidance of choice is still a choice that also will carry consequences. These choices cover every aspect of life, from health and lifestyle

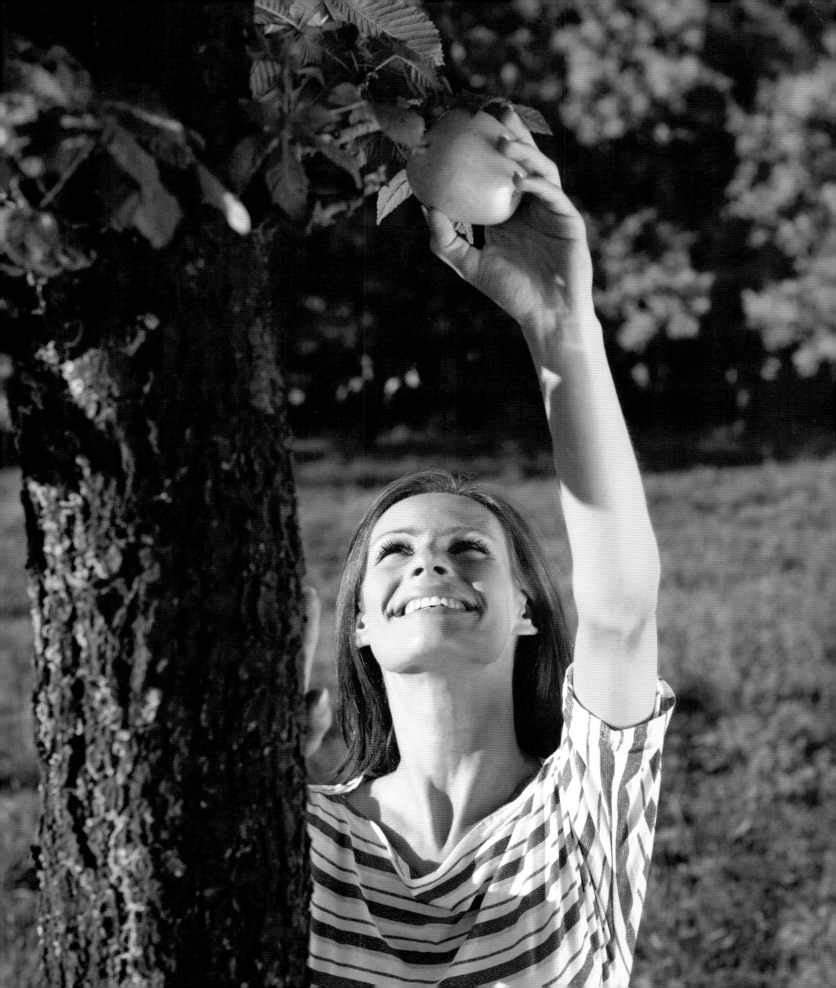

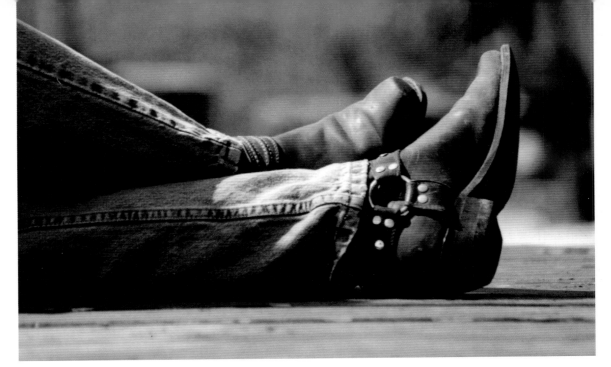

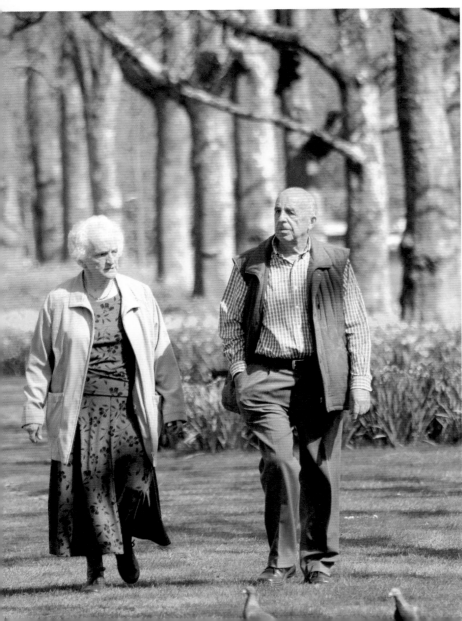

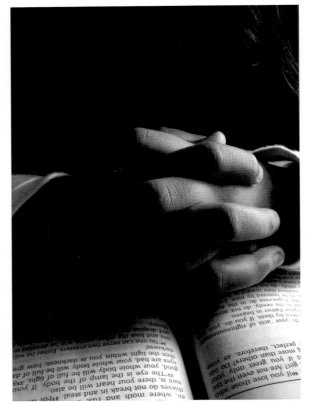

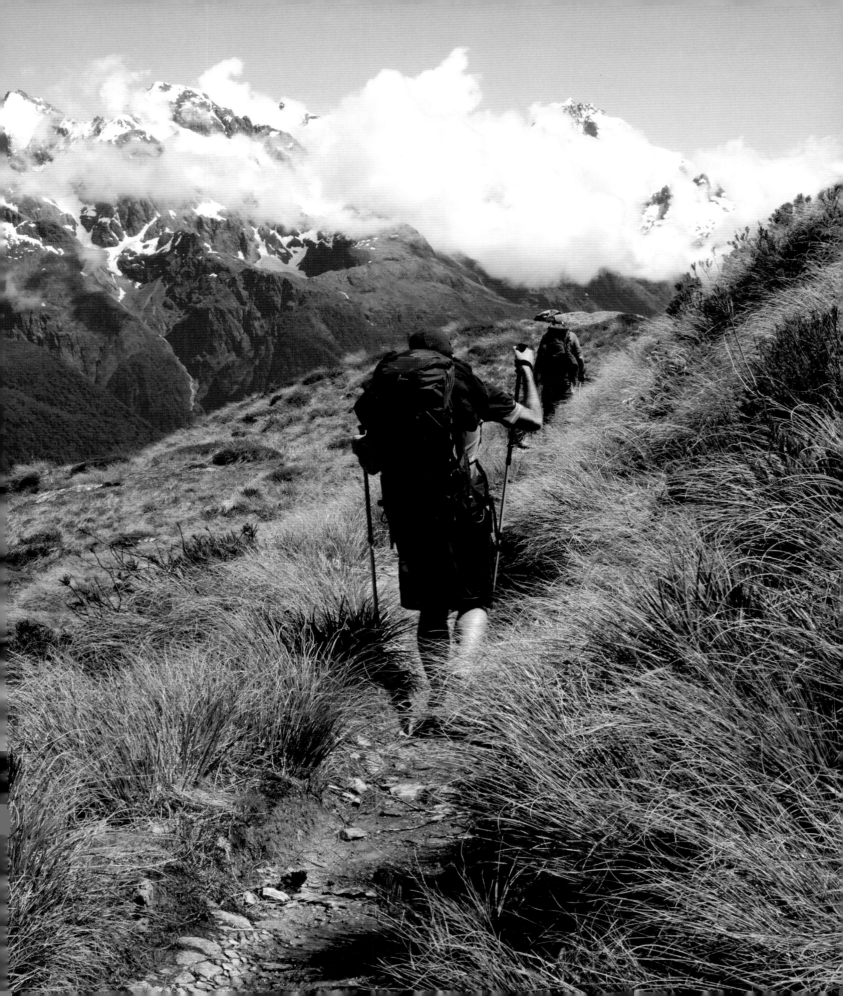

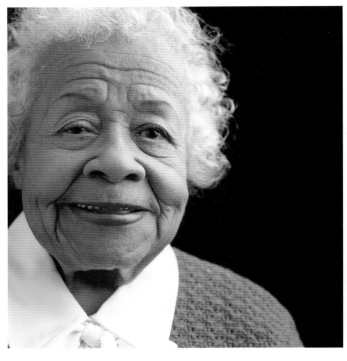
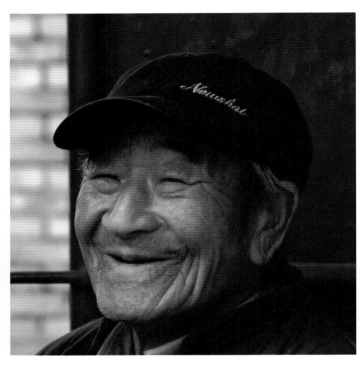
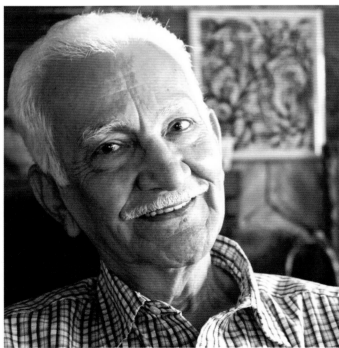
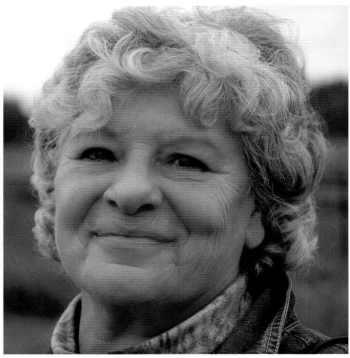

issues to those involving integrity, spirituality, and relationships.

BASIS FOR INFORMED CHOICES

It's tempting to make choices based on personal bias rather than on evidence and high-quality studies. We need to recognize that there are differences in the quality, consistency, numbers, importance, and generalizability of studies. Such awareness can temper our rigidity, help us to weigh the evidence, and ultimately influence our choices.

In 2010 the Dietary Guideline Advisory Committee of the United States Department of Agriculture and the Department of Health and Human Services recommended that studies be classified by the body of evidence supporting their conclusions. They designated as strong those studies in which the quality, consistency, numbers, importance, and generalizability were of the highest order; moderate where such factors were less conclusive, and limited for those of weak design. Such choices and practices based on this type of information are called "evidence-based."

Living in conformity with cultural traditions of forebears often has gone on for centuries, with the reasons for certain behaviors and beliefs hidden in the mists of time. Many practices have absolutely no basis in fact. It's not difficult to debunk the benefits of practices such as applying cattle dung to a newborn's umbilicus, but possibly harder to argue convincingly with a cultural belief that a woman should not bathe for a month after giving birth.

In the first half of the nineteenth century, "health reformers" developed a litany of health laws based on scant evidence. Fortunately, today a wealth of evidence can guide us in making choices. Principles of balance and moderation, with the avoidance of harmful substances, will pay dividends in the health of temperate and informed people.

One of the early classic studies on lifestyle and health was published in 1972. Drs. Nedra Belloc and Lester Breslow, from the U. S. Department of Public Health in Berkeley, California, were among the first researchers to present convincing answers on lifestyle habits that promote longevity. In their study of 6,928 adult residents of Alameda County, California, they found that some lifestyle habits influenced longevity:[2]

1. ▶ Adequate sleep (7 to 8 hours per night)

2. ▶ No eating between meals

3. ▶ A nutritious daily breakfast

4. ▶ The maintenance of the recommended weight for one's height, bone structure, and age (BMI, or Body Mass Index)

5. ▶ Regular physical activity

6. ▶ The nonuse of tobacco

7. ▶ A reduction in the use of alcoholic beverages (the GC Health Department advocates abstinence)

In a nine-year follow-up they showed that the more of these seven habits a person regularly followed, the greater their chance of longevity. Of the group following all seven habits, only 5.5 percent of men and 5.3 percent of women died before the end of the nine-year period; whereas in the group that followed only three of the seven habits, 20 percent of the men and 12.3 percent of the women died.[3]

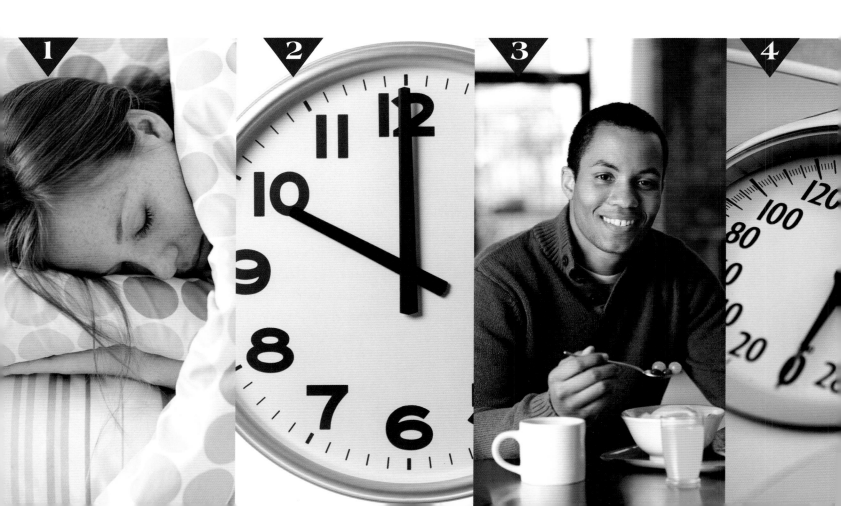

The more of these seven habits a person regularly followed, the greater their chance of longevity.

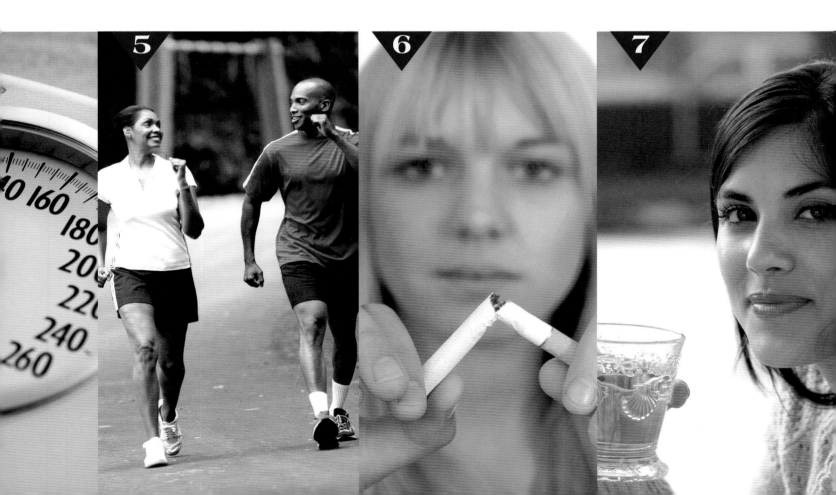

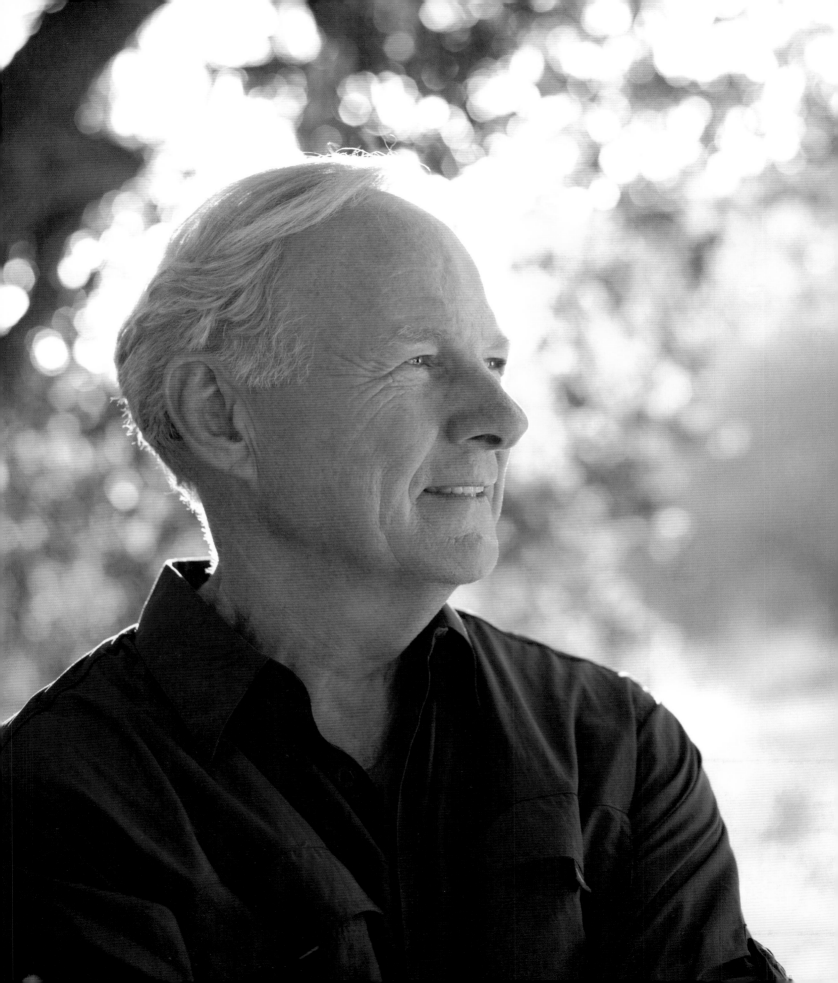

STAY OBJECTIVE

Even when clearly intentional, freely made, and informed, choices and decisions are not always easy to make, particularly when trying to maintain objectivity. So keep in mind the following:

■ Get the facts and weigh them on the scale of common sense.

■ When possible, don't make choices in the midst of highly stressful situations, when it's more difficult to think clearly.

■ Watch out for the distortion your emotional state can bring to decision-making. Anger, depression, and elation can influence decisions.

■ Don't assume things. Just because sugar tastes good, it doesn't mean it's good for you. Similarly, something that tastes bad isn't necessarily improving your health.

■ Beware of wishful thinking. Don't overlook that lump because you wish it would go away. Don't think you can walk a mile to get rid of the calories in a piece of coconut cream pie.

■ Be careful where you get your health advice. Quackery is still thriving in a multitude of guises.

■ Trust in intelligence; choose the smart over the unwise, the good over the bad. Also beware of the dead-end path that takes you nowhere.

■ Choose to do what you can do, not what you want to do. Our wants are often beyond us, and they are so many.

A GIFT FROM GOD

Adventists see good health as a gift from our Creator God. The proper "preventive maintenance" reduces risk and leads to a happier, healthier, and longer life. No one lives forever, though, and even the best maintenance cannot guarantee a disease-free life.

Recent scientific studies also indicate the importance of spirituality to mental health. With anxiety disorders being the most prevalent of the emotional disorders, spiritual exercises such as Bible reading and meditation on the life of Christ can bring great peace—one of the ingredients of mental health.

For some, the quality of life is more important than its duration. There are chronically ill people who are

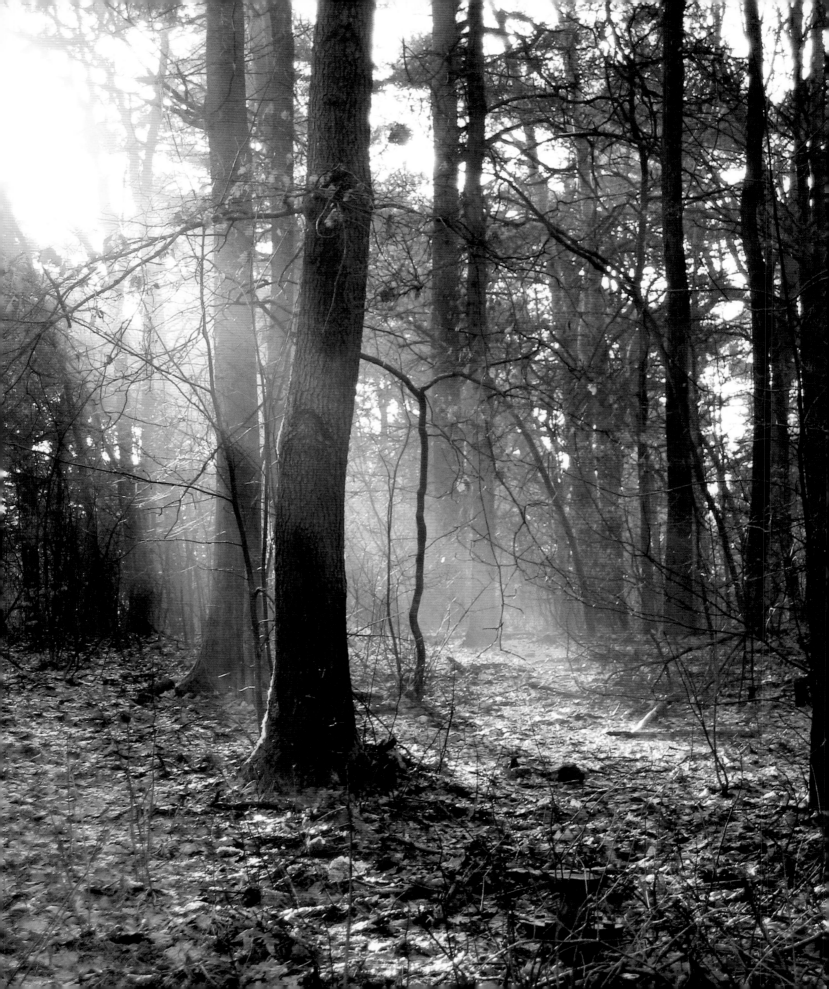

happy and content, because they intentionally have chosen to make the best of their situation. Similarly, many who are perfectly healthy physically may nurture a negative mind-set that destroys their equanimity. People choose their "attitude," and this affects the way they relate to triumphs or disasters—and many situations in between.

One area of choice, of course, is what we believe. Science does not illuminate all aspects of life, and so people live in or by a system of beliefs. Some call this "faith." Many—including me, as the writer—have chosen to believe in God as our Creator and heavenly Father, even though we cannot see or touch Him. Having chosen to believe, a huge amount of supportive evidence may be amassed to support this belief. At its core, however, it's a choice—the most important choice any person can make, because it's only by developing and maintaining a close walk with our Lord that we will truly obtain optimal whole health and know the joy of living well, both here and throughout eternity.

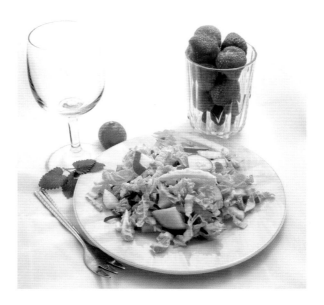

Celebrating Choices: Life-Application Questions

Take the time to consider these questions and apply what you are learning to your life.

I What choices am I making, consciously or unconsciously, that are not based on evidence? How do these choices affect my use of time; my health; my relationships at work, at home, or with God? What are my reasons for making these choices? In what ways are they influenced by my culture or my emotions? Is it because I wish to please myself? Or am I being careless? Do I accept as evidence anything and everything I read on the Internet? Does just one anecdote convince me of the "right" thing to do?

2 What negative choices have other people made that influenced the trajectory of my life? How have I reacted to those circumstances? What freedoms do I enjoy that allow me to choose to change the direction in which I am heading? How can I choose to improve my attitude even under less-than-ideal circumstances?

3 How many of the seven habits that influence longevity am I practicing regularly? Am I getting sufficient sleep, exercising regularly, avoiding tobacco and alcohol, eating a good breakfast and nothing in between meals? Is my Body Mass Index (BMI) within recommended limits? (See www.nhlbisupport.com/bmi for a handy calculator.) Which ones will I choose to introduce into my lifestyle today? Could I improve on any of the seven?

GROUP DISCUSSION

4 Chris went out to a business dinner after a long day at work. Before leaving he was accused of something he had not done. He later tells a friend that after a few drinks he relaxed and decided to resign his job, move to a different city, and look for work there. What influenced his hasty decision? What did he forget to do? How should he have acted in this situation?

5 Discuss recent poor choices group members have made including the pressures that may have influenced those choices, such as stress, anger, and depression. Were decisions made late at night or after a heavy meal or a long day of work? How can we avoid making choices when in these types of emotional states? How important is it to ask for divine guidance? Is there a particular time of day that is better for decision-making? In what ways does making wise small choices help with making big decisions? What other things help when making a big decision?

6 What choices are important to make regarding our relationship with our Creator, who graciously gives us the freedom to choose? How can we increase our awareness of His love and His interest in our choices? Do we need to spend more time learning about Him in His Word or in nature? Do we have to cultivate conversation with Him in prayer? How can we continue to build supportive evidence for our faith?

What choices am I making, consciously or unconsciously, that are not based on evidence?

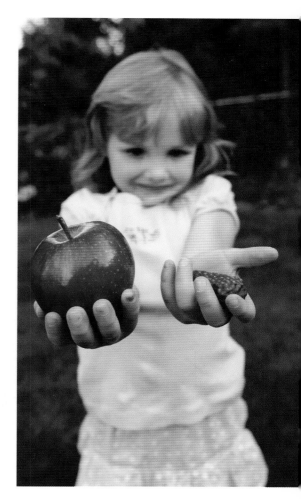

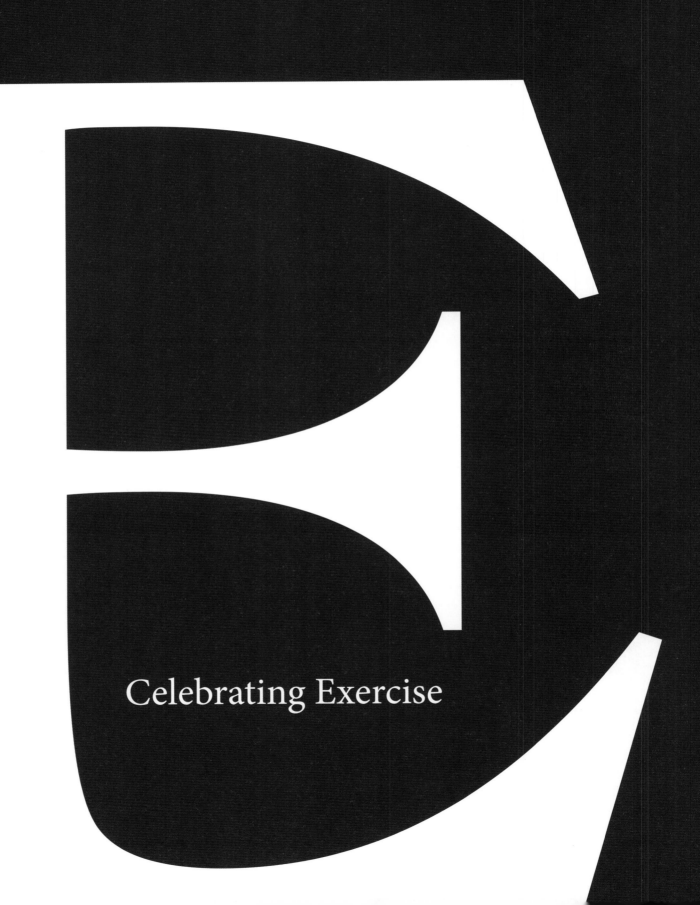

Celebrating Exercise

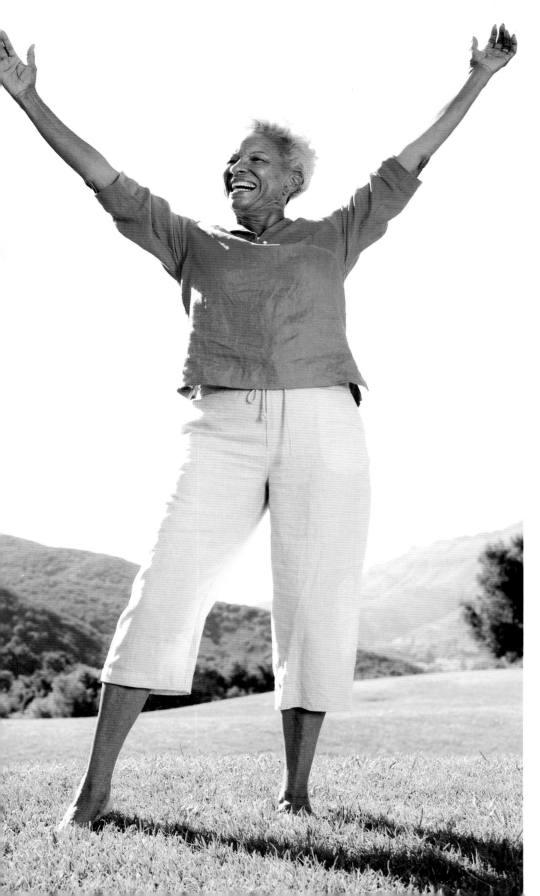

At age 91 Grace was still active playing tennis, lifting weights, and walking. Fifty-one years before, however, at the age of 40, her condition had been very different. Grace's spine was badly injured during a ski accident that occurred at the time, and as the years passed her back pain intensified. Her physician told her that he couldn't do much to help her because she was "too old." Grace later was diagnosed with emphysema and had difficulty breathing. She tired easily and at one point feared that she would never be able to climb stairs again. The doctor offered her no hope of improvement.

Grace, however, had a strong will to recover and decided to try an exercise program offered at a local medical center. For six weeks she worked out three times a week, two to three hours a day. She lifted weights, walked

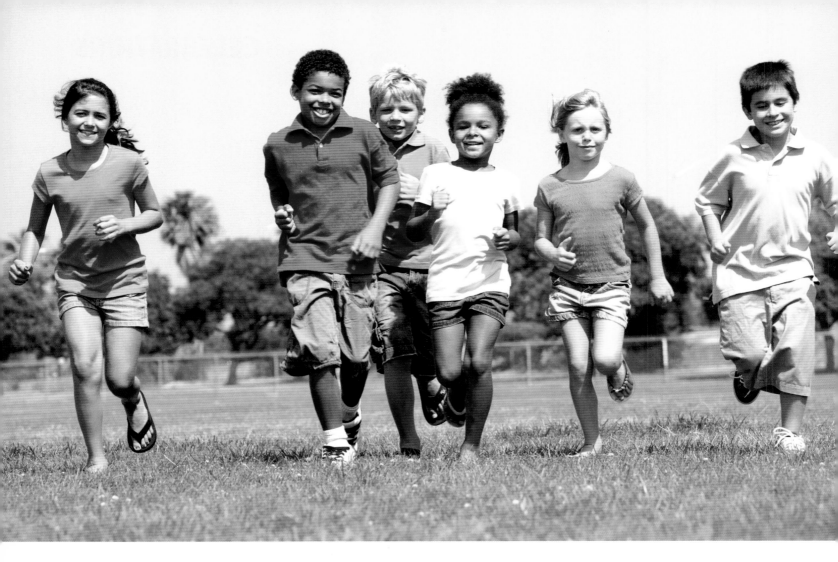

on the treadmill, rode the stationary bicycle, and did breathing exercises. Even when she was in pain and didn't feel like doing anything, she didn't quit. Eventually, her breathing improved and the back pain disappeared. She was able to walk reasonable distances—and had energy to spare! Her doctor told her that he had never seen such progress in anyone her age. Grace attributes her health improvement to exercise.[1]

BENEFITS OF PHYSICAL EXERCISE

Exercise is a form of physical activity that is planned, structured, repetitive, and performed with the goal of improving health and fitness. So although all exercise is physical activity, not all physical activity is exercise.

Regular exercise is not only a preventive measure; it also works to maintain health at its best. Studies clearly demonstrate that participating in regular physical activity provides many health benefits. The Physical Activity Guidelines for Americans (PAGA) Advisory Committee, comprising 13 leading experts in the field of exercise science and public health, summarizes the benefits of exercise in the adjacent table. [2]

HEALTH BENEFITS ASSOCIATED WITH REGULAR PHYSICAL ACTIVITY

CHILDREN AND ADOLESCENTS

Strong Evidence

Improved cardiorespiratory and muscular fitness

Improved bone health

Improved cardiovascular and metabolic health biomarkers

Favorable body composition

Moderate Evidence

Reduced symptoms of depression

ADULTS AND OLDER ADULTS

Strong Evidence

Lower risk of early death

Lower risk of coronary heart disease

Lower risk of stroke

Lower risk of high blood pressure

Lower risk of adverse blood lipid profile

Lower risk of type 2 diabetes

Lower risk of metabolic syndrome

Lower risk of colon cancer

Lower risk of breast cancer

Prevention of weight gain

Weight loss, particularly when combined with reduced calorie intake

Improved cardiorespiratory and muscular fitness

Prevention of falls

Reduced depression

Better cognitive function (for older adults)

Moderate to Strong Evidence

Better functional health (for older adults)

Reduced abdominal obesity

Moderate Evidence

Lower risk of hip fracture

Lower risk of lung cancer

Lower risk of endometrial cancer

Weight maintenance after weight loss

Increased bone density

Improved sleep quality

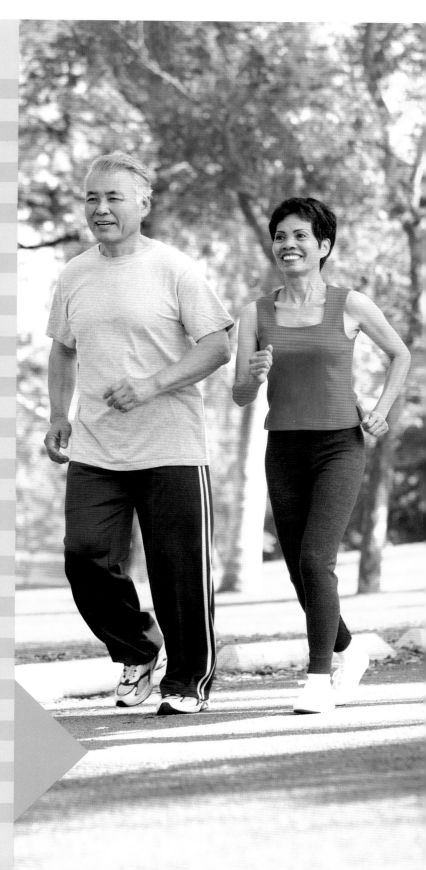

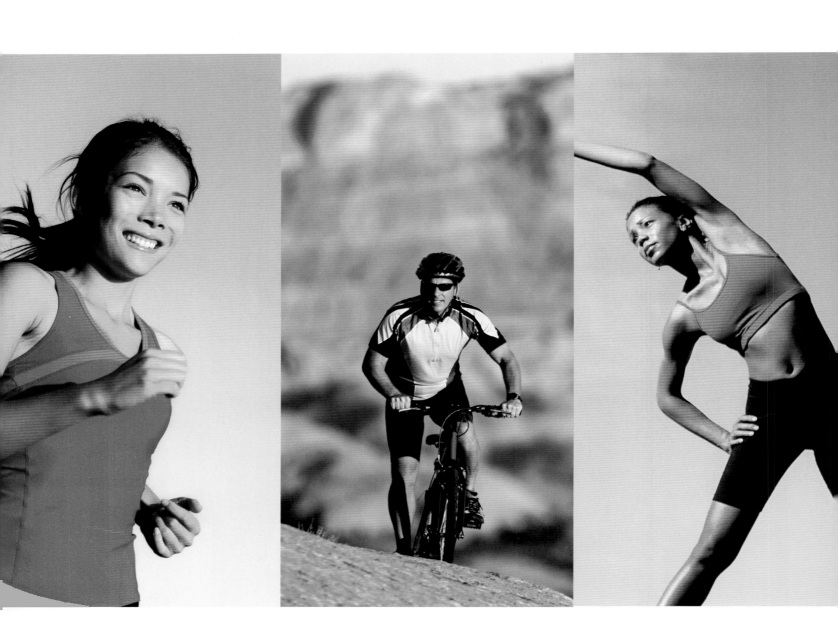

Exercise is a form of physical activity that is planned, structured, repetitive, and performed with the goal of improving health and fitness.

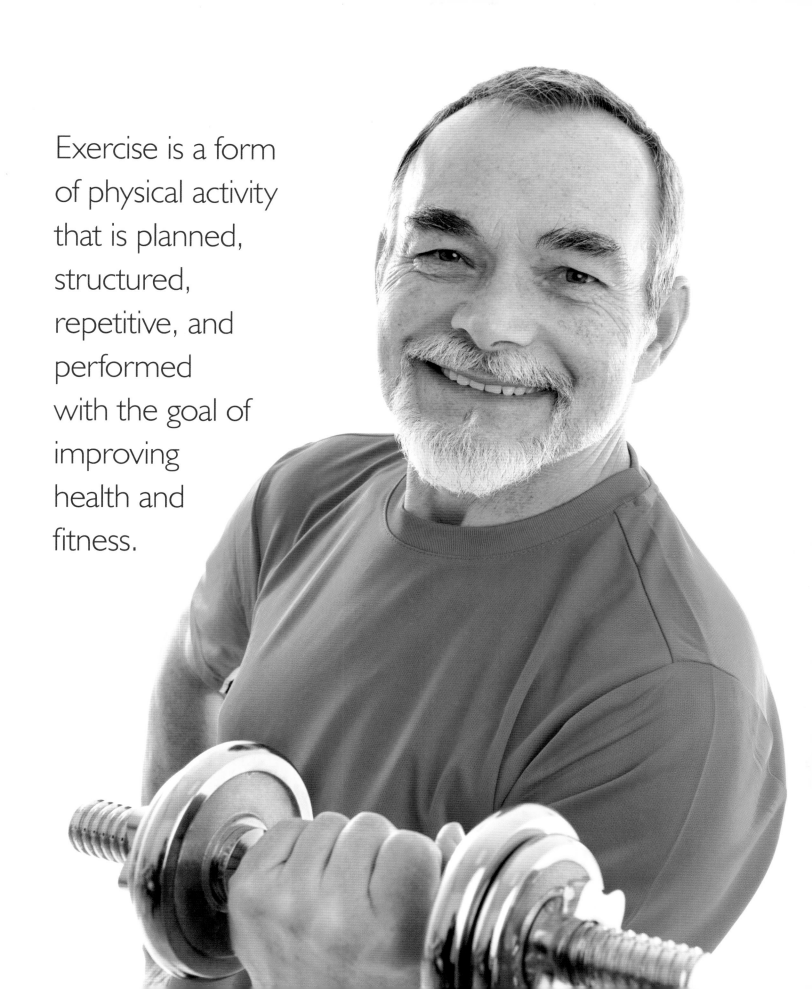

Studies show that people who are physically active for approximately seven hours a week have a 40-percent lower risk of dying prematurely than those who are active for fewer than 30 minutes a week. There's even substantially lower risk of premature death when people do two and a half hours of at least moderate-intensity aerobic physical activity a week.

CARDIOVASCULAR DISEASE

Heart disease and stroke are two of the leading causes of death worldwide. Studies show that a significant reduction in the risk of cardiovascular disease occurs at activity levels equivalent to two and a half hours a week of moderate-intensity physical activity. The evidence is strong that greater amounts of physical activity up to one hour per day result in further reductions in risk of cardiovascular disease.

MUSCULOSKELETAL HEALTH

The decline in bone density during aging can be slowed with regular physical activity beginning at one and a half hours a week and continuing up to five hours a week. Research studies of physical activity to prevent hip fracture show that participating in two to five hours of physical activity per week of at least moderate intensity is associated with reduced risk.

METABOLIC HEALTH

Metabolic Syndrome is a condition in which people have a combination of high blood pressure, a large waistline (abdominal obesity), an adverse blood lipid profile (low levels of high-density lipoprotein [HDL] cholesterol, raised triglycerides), and impaired glucose tolerance. Studies have shown that people with metabolic syndrome respond to persistent, regular physical activity; a restrictive diet; and appropriate medications.[3] Other studies show that those who regularly engage in at least two to two and a half hours a week of moderate-intensity aerobic activity have a lower risk of developing type 2 diabetes than do inactive people.

OBESITY AND ENERGY BALANCE

Overweight and obesity occur when calories ingested through food and beverages are more than calories used. Research shows that within the space of a year it's possible to achieve weight stability through two and a half to five hours per week of walking at a pace of about four miles per hour. Such physical activity is a critical factor in determining whether a person can maintain a healthy body weight, lose excess body weight, or maintain successful weight.

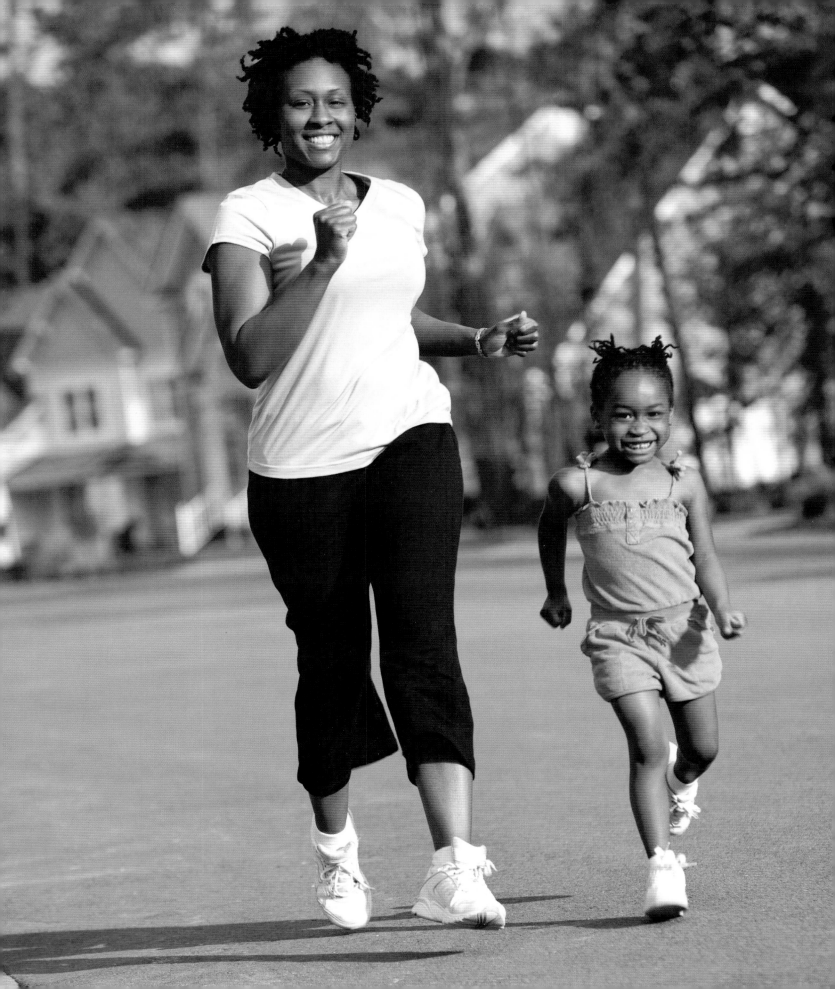

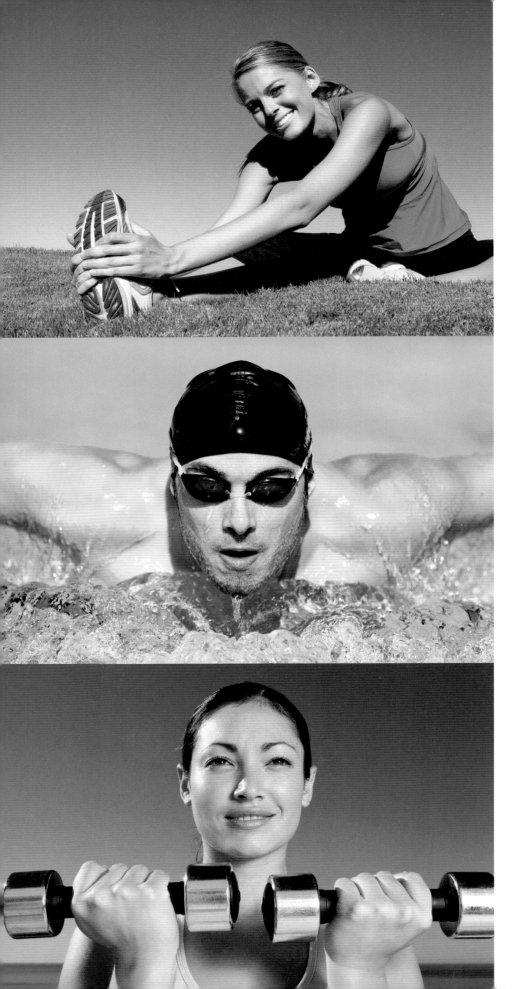

Health benefits of physical activity far outweigh the risk of adverse events for almost everyone. Adults with chronic disabilities should consult their health-care provider about the types and amounts of activity appropriate for them. As long as the activity is within one's ability, it should be safe. In other words, if you want to postpone your funeral, exercise regularly!

THREE TYPES OF PHYSICAL ACTIVITIES

Physical exercises are generally grouped into three types[4] and have different effects on the body:

■ Flexibility exercises, such as stretching, improve the range of motion of muscles and joints.[5]

■ Aerobic exercises, such as cycling, swimming, walking, skipping rope, rowing, running, hiking, or playing tennis, focus on increasing cardiovascular endurance;[6] however, weight-bearing aerobic exercise, such as walking, climbing, and jogging, increases bone density.

■ Resistance exercises, such as weight training, increase muscle strength[7] and lower or prevent bone loss associated with menopause.[8]

FOUR LEVELS OF
PHYSICAL ACTIVITY

The 2008 PAGA Advisory Committee report provides the basis for dividing the amount of weekly aerobic physical activity for adults into four levels:

1 Inactive—no additional activity beyond baseline (basic routine activities)

2 Low—some exercise, up to 150 minutes a week

3 Medium—exercise 150 to 300 minutes a week

4 High—exercise more than 300 minutes a week

These categories provide a rule of thumb for how the total amount of physical activity is related to health benefits. Low amounts of activity provide some benefit; medium amounts provide substantial benefit; and high amounts provide even greater benefit. If a person has not been exercising regularly, it's important to obtain health clearance from a physician before embarking on such a program.

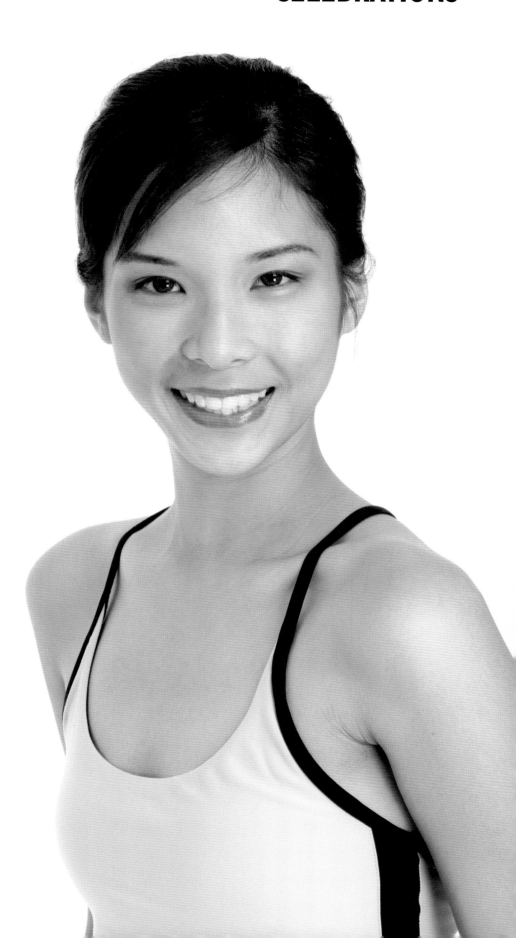

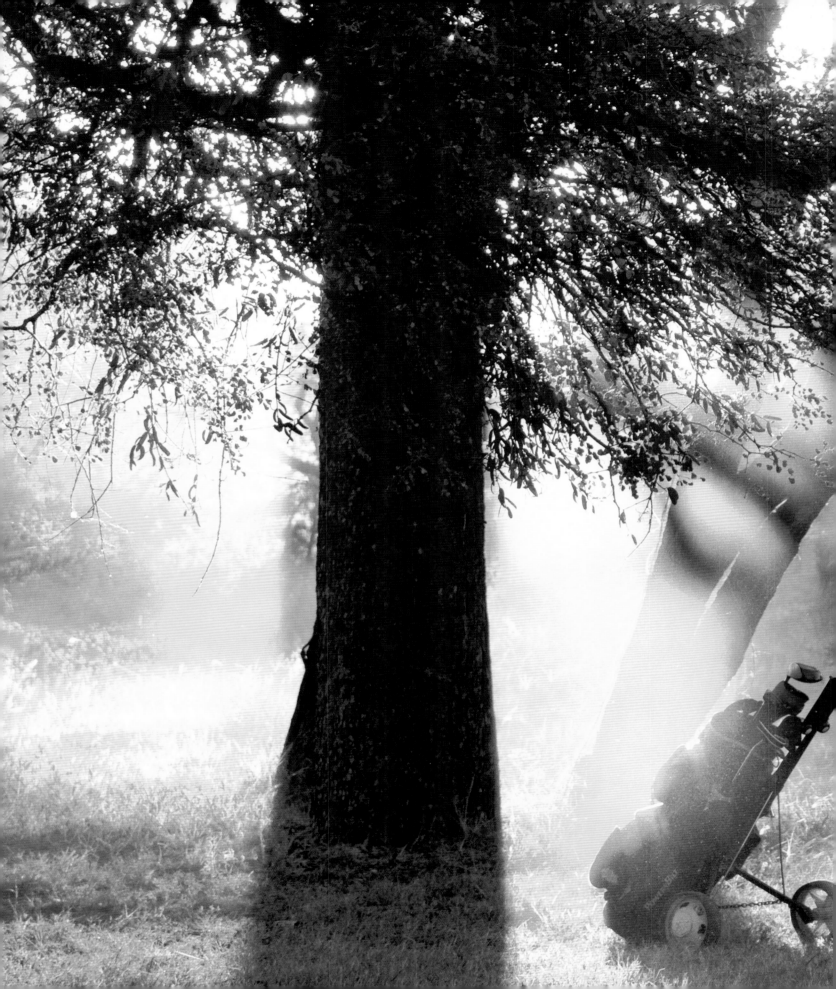

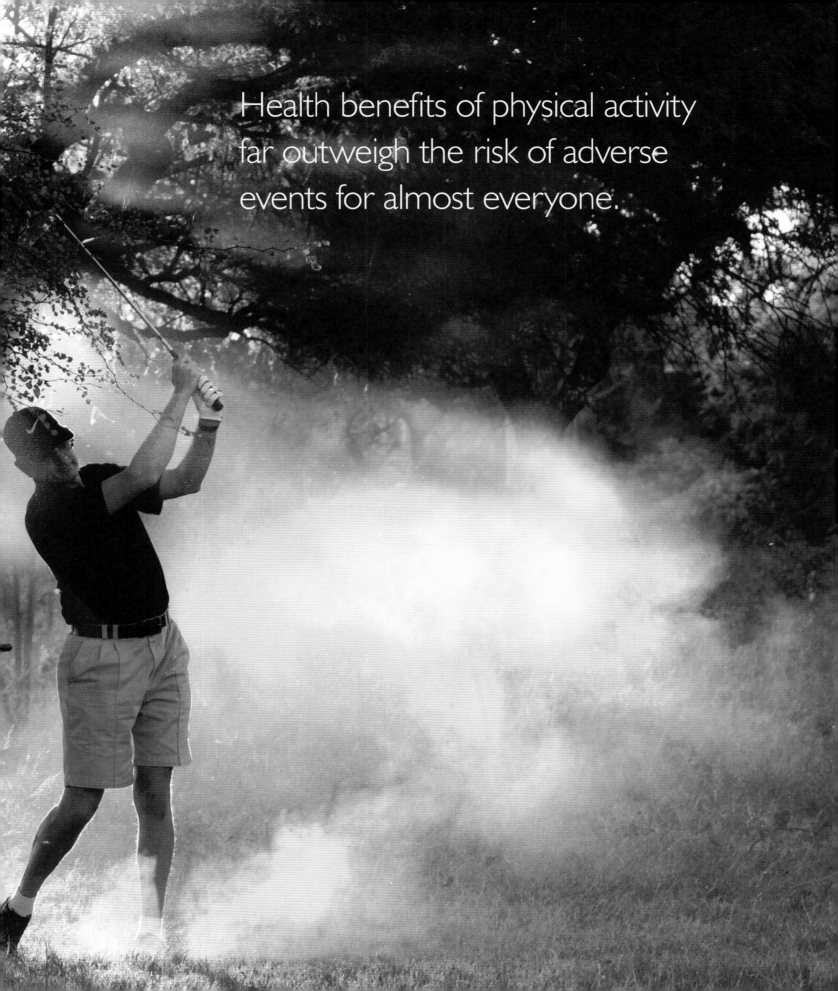

Health benefits of physical activity far outweigh the risk of adverse events for almost everyone.

PHYSICAL ACTIVITY GUIDELINES

The 2008 Physical Activity Guidelines for Americans recommend that a person accumulate two and a half hours a week in various activities. This would be applicable worldwide. Examples of aerobic physical activities and intensities are shown in the following table:

Moderate Intensity
Walking briskly (three miles per hour or faster, but not racewalking)
Water aerobics
Bicycling slower than 10 miles per hour
Tennis (doubles)
General gardening

Vigorous Intensity
Racewalking, jogging, or running
Swimming laps
Tennis (singles)
Bicycling 10 miles per hour or faster
Skipping rope
Heavy gardening (continuous digging or hoeing, with heart rate increases)
Hiking uphill or with a heavy backpack

How do we know the intensity of our exercise? As a rule of thumb, a person doing moderate-intensity aerobic activity can maintain a comfortable conversation during the activity. A person doing vigorous-intensity activity cannot say more than a few words without pausing for a breath.

Health benefits have not yet been proved for activities such as stretching, warming up, or cooling down, but they often are used in physical activity programs.

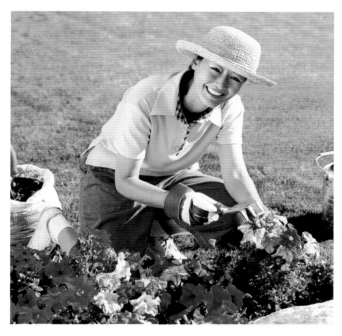

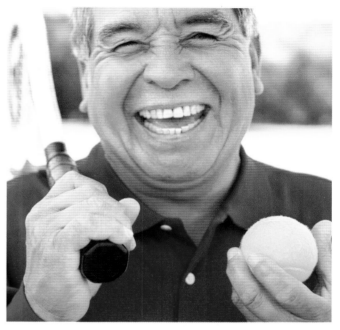

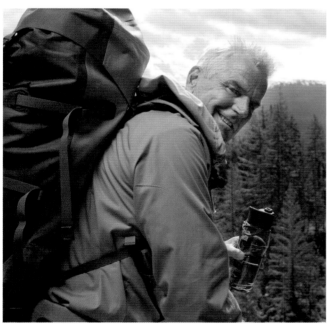

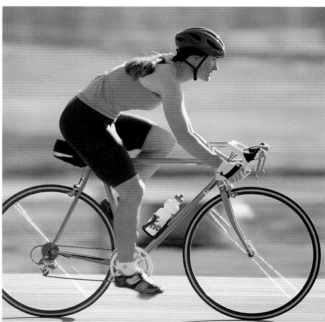

SAFE WHILE ACTIVE

Although physical activity has many health benefits, injuries and other adverse events do sometimes occur. The most common injuries affect the musculoskeletal system (bones, joints, muscles, ligaments, and tendons). Others problems, such as overheating and dehydration, may occur during activity. The good news is that scientific evidence strongly shows that appropriate physical activity is safe for almost everyone, and that the health benefits of physical activity far outweigh the risks.

THE BEST PHYSICAL ACTIVITY

The current Physical Activity Guidelines for Americans encourage a person to accumulate at least two and a half hours a week in moderate-intensity physical activity, such as brisk walking. Dr. Kenneth Cooper, of *Aerobics* fame, promotes brisk walking rather

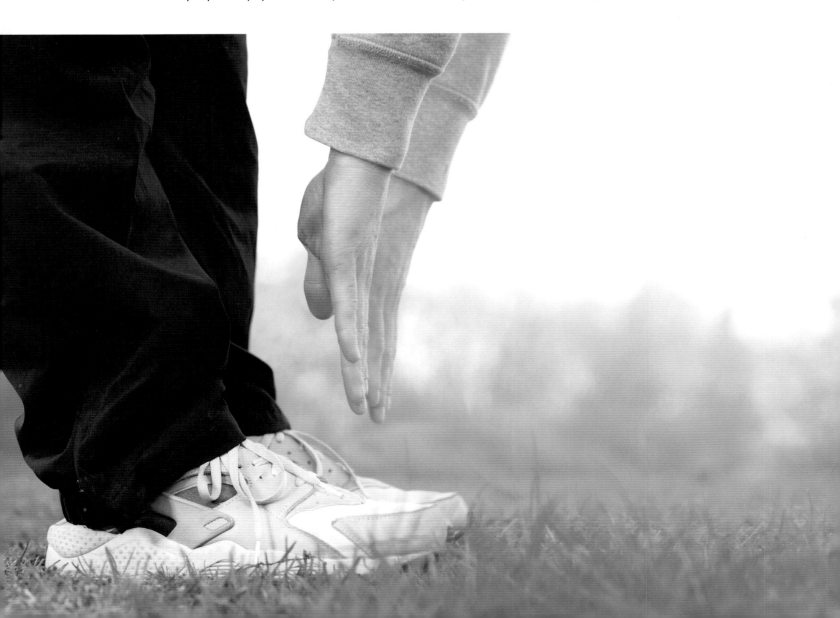

than running or jogging. Walking appeals to many because it can be done almost any time or place. It's fun, convenient, inexpensive, and can be enjoyed alone or with friends. It requires no special equipment. Comfortable walking shoes and clothing are all that is needed. Brisk walking results in minimal injuries while exercising most muscles and systems of the body. It stimulates the release of endorphins, which elevate the mood and improve outlook on life.

More than 150 years ago Ellen G. White said, "Walking, in all cases where it is possible, is the best exercise, because in walking, all the muscles are brought into action."[9]

PROPER TRAINING CLOTHING

While exercising one should wear lightweight garments that offer maximum freedom of movement and are appropriate to climatic conditions. When exercising in an urban area, use brightly colored garments and reflector materials for safety.

Exercise generates heat, so it's better to dress in layers that can be removed as soon as one starts perspiring. If it's very cold, consider wearing a face mask or scarf to warm the air before it enters the lungs. A hat or headband will protect the ears, which are vulnerable to frostbite.

It's vital to wear protective gear, such as helmets, wrist guards, and knee guards, when engaging in physical activities that carry risk of injury, including bicycling, skateboarding, and rollerblading.

PROPER TRAINING SHOES

Feet bear the weight of the whole body, therefore it's important that shoes be comfortable, well-fitting, and supportive. Look for athletic shoes with absorbent cushioning, appropriate arch support, a solid and snug heel cup, flexibility, breathability, and good lacing so you can adjust tightness without pinching your feet.

EXERCISING FAITH

As regular aerobic exercise helps us live better, so it is with the exercise of faith. We can trust God to lead our lives according to His loving prescription for health.

He gives power to the weak, and to those who have no might He increases strength. Even the youths shall faint and be weary, and the young men shall utterly fall, but those who wait on the Lord shall renew their strength; they shall mount up with wings like eagles, they shall run and not be weary, they shall walk and not faint (Isa. 40:29-31, NKJV).

Celebrating Exercise: Life-Application Questions

Take the time to consider these questions and apply what you are learning to your life.

1 What are the most attractive benefits of regular exercise? How can I live longer with better cognitive function and lower my risk of getting cancer, cardiovascular disease, or diabetes? How does exercise offer better quality of life, less depression, ease of movement, and optimum body mass? As I look at my family history are there benefits of exercise that could prevent the adverse history being repeated in my life? Am I going to make the choice to exercise with these goals as motivating factors?

2 How much exercise am I currently getting per week? What level of exercise am I achieving? Do I need to choose to exercise for longer periods each day, or can I increase the level of activity? What activity can I do along with exercises such as walking to maximize my use of time? Should I use the time for personal growth, possibly spiritual, by listening to an audio version of the Bible or devotional books? What benefits would come from exercising with friends? Would I be able to maintain some long-distance relationships by talking on the phone while doing moderate-intensity aerobic exercise?

3 How can I become better motivated to exercise regularly? What types of exercise achieve flexibility, cardiovascular fitness, and improved bone health? Which of the three types will I start today? When will I include the next type of exercise?

GROUP DISCUSSION

4 The children of Margaret's neighbor have a problem with their weight, and Margaret is worried that they are at risk for diabetes. She wants to give them a gift at Christmas. What should she get that would make exercise fun for them?

5 Are there others, such as our spouses, who need to be encouraged to exercise? Discuss ways to do that, such as making time to walk together, thereby adding more bonding time with our marriage partner or other loved one.

6 What is the best clothing and shoes for exercise activities? What improves safety when exercising in a busy city, at night, or during winter?

7 It's sometimes difficult to choose to exercise on a daily basis. How can we obtain spiritual strength to make this a priority in our life?

How can I become better motivated to exercise regularly?

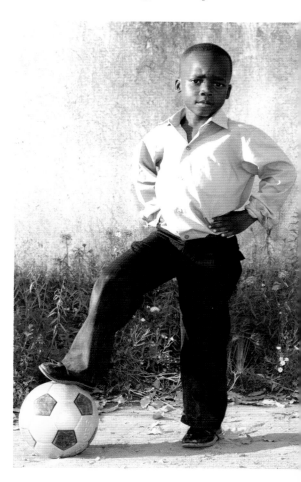

Celebrating Liquids

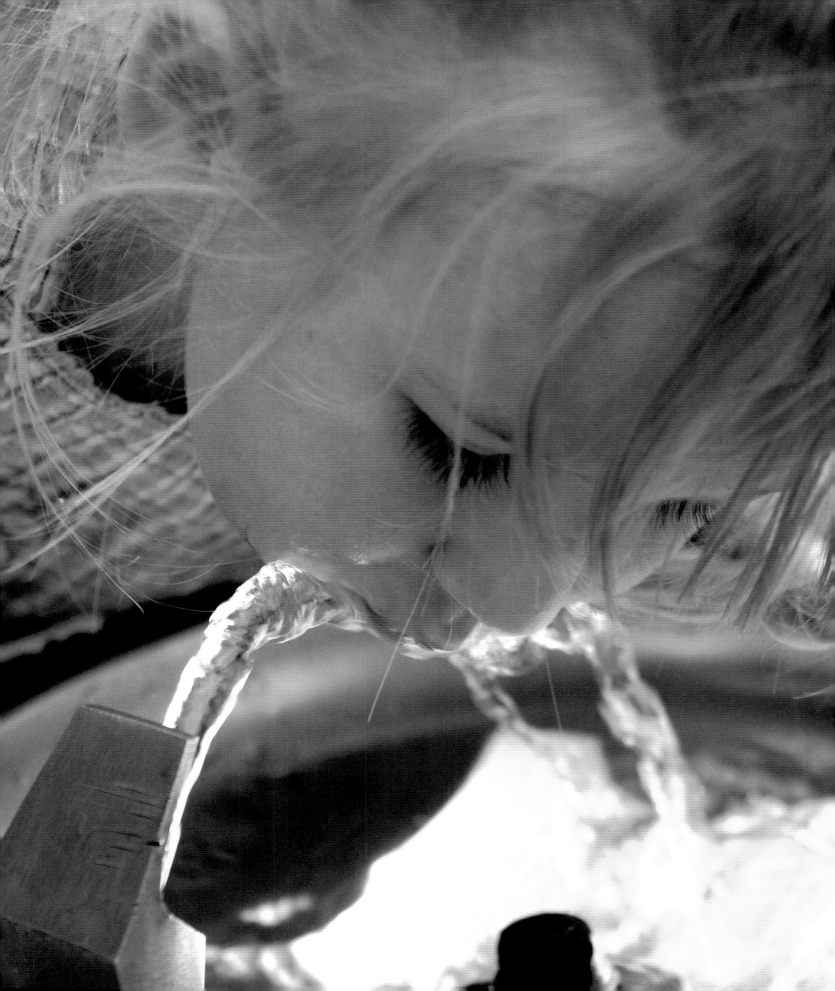

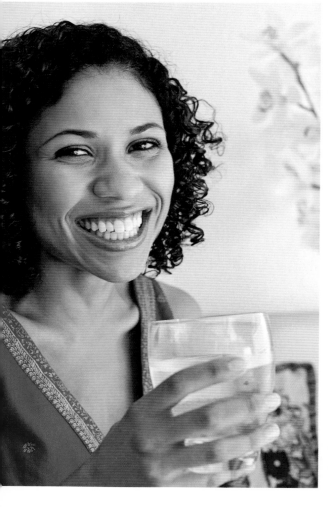

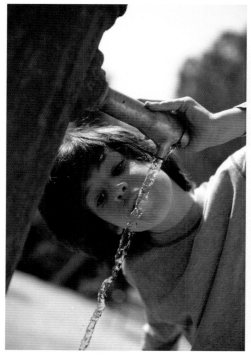

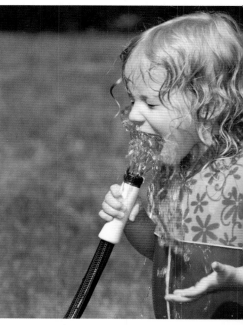

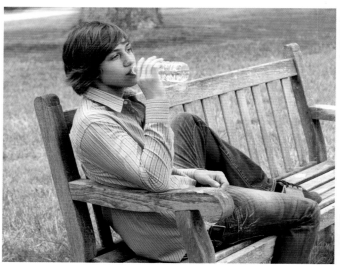

L i Ming was a re-tired woman who enjoyed working in her garden. Even the unusual heat wave that hit her region one summer didn't deter her from tending her flowers and other plants. The temperature rose above 100 degrees Fahrenheit, and the humidity teetered at 90 percent. On the third day of these record-breaking temperatures, Li Ming called her daughter, Kim, but Li Ming sounded confused on the phone. Kim became alarmed and rushed to Li Ming's house, where she found her mother lying on the kitchen floor unconscious. Apparently, Li Ming's large fan wasn't enough to fight the effects of the heat and humidity, and she suffered heat stroke—which can be life threatening.[1]

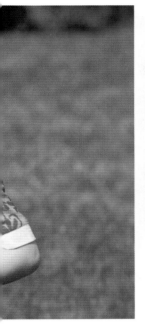

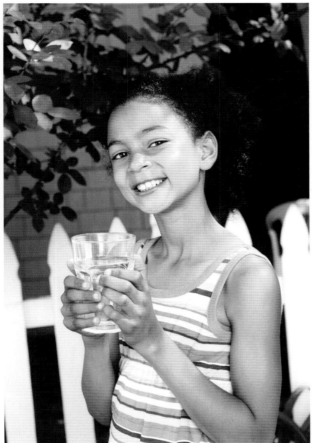

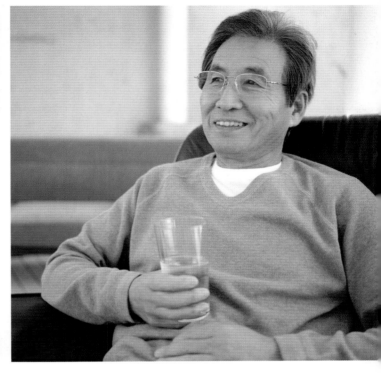

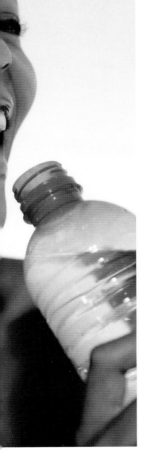

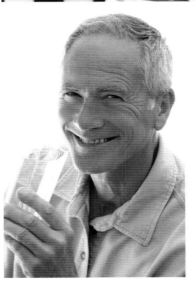

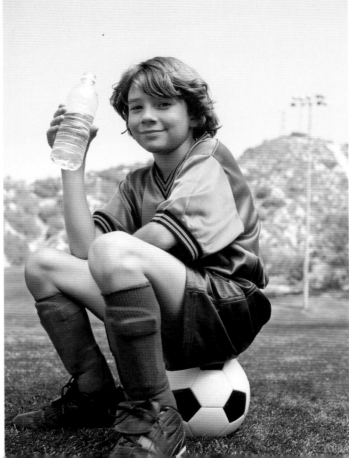

One can lower the risk of heat-related illness, such as heat stroke, by drinking plenty of liquids, particularly water and fruit and vegetable juices. Next to air, water is the most vital element needed for survival. By weight, a newborn infant is approximately 75 percent water, and an adult about 70 percent. A man weighing 198 pounds has about 138 pounds of water in his body.

The gray matter of the brain is approximately 85 percent water, blood is 83 percent water, muscles are about 75 percent water, and even hard marrow bones are 20 to 25 percent water.[2] Almost every cell and tissue of the body not only contains water but is continually bathed in fluid and requires water to perform its functions.

Water, the liquid of life, is a medium in which metabolism takes place. It is:

the transport system within the body

a lubricant for movement

the facilitator of digestion

the prime transporter of waste via the kidneys

a temperature regulator

a major constituent of the circulating blood

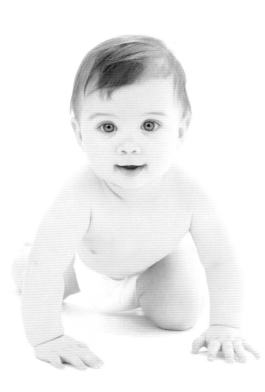

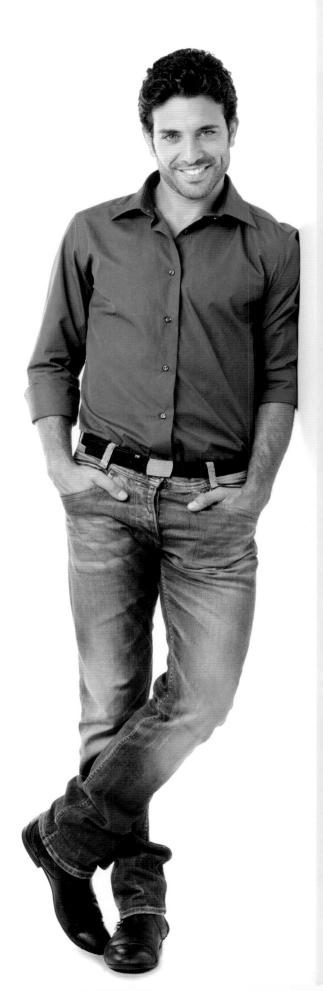

About two thirds of the water our body requires come from ingested liquid, about one third from our food, and a small amount of liquid is synthesized during food metabolism. Fruits and vegetables generally have higher water content than other food groups. Examples include:

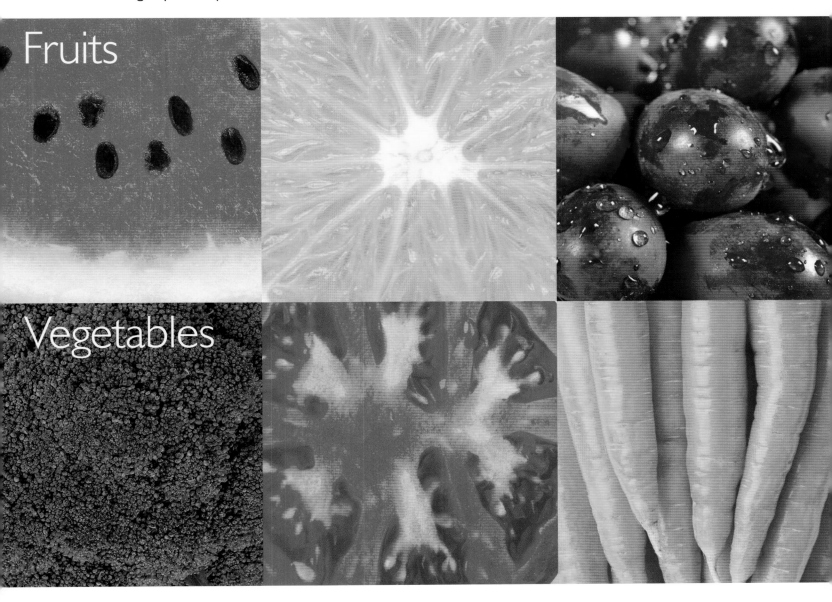

Fruits

Vegetables

Apricots Watermelon Papaya	Spinach Bell Peppers Lettuce
Citrus Strawberries Apples	Carrots Cucumbers Squash
Grapes Cherries	Broccoli Celery Tomatoes

Ideally, the body maintains a balance between the amount of water lost each day and the amount taken in to replace it. The amount of daily water lost depends on climatic conditions and physical activities, as shown in the adjacent table.

The table shows that sweat is excreted 50 times quicker under conditions of prolonged heavy exercise compared to low activity in normal temperatures. The average human excretes a total of some 2,300 milliliters of water daily during low activity at normal temperature, and 6,600 milliliters in prolonged heavy exercise.[3]

Daily Loss of Water in Milliliters Per Day of an Average Human Body at Normal Temperature

	Low Activity	Prolonged Heavy Exercise
Insensible (invisible) loss from skin	350	350
Insensible (invisible) loss from lungs	350	650
Sweat	100	5000
Feces	100	100
Urine	1400	500
Total Output	**2300**	**6600**

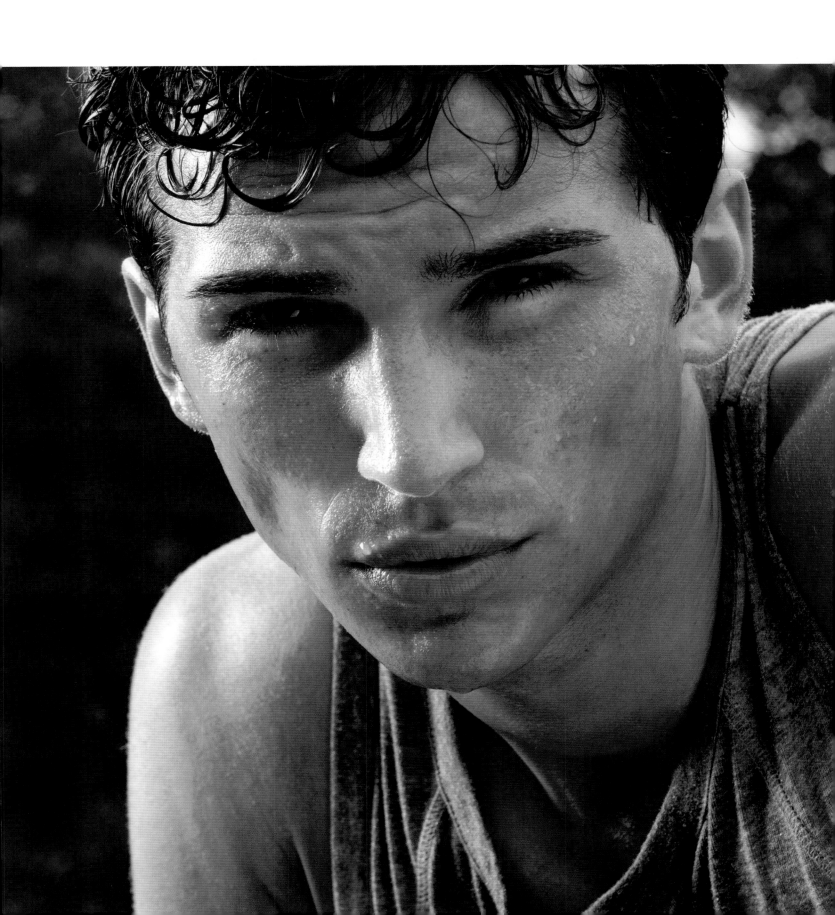

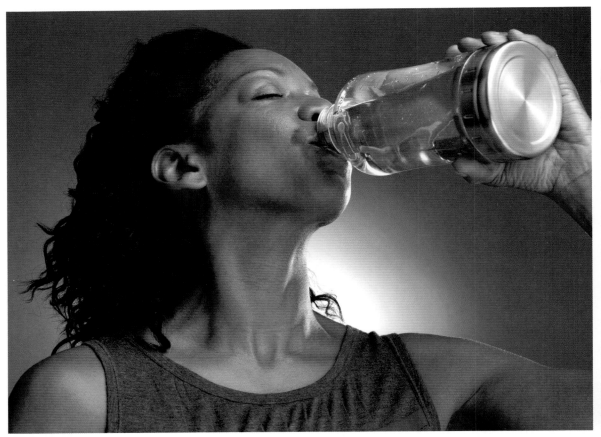
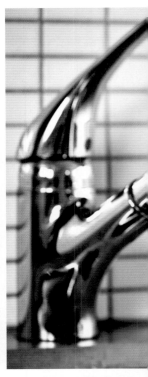
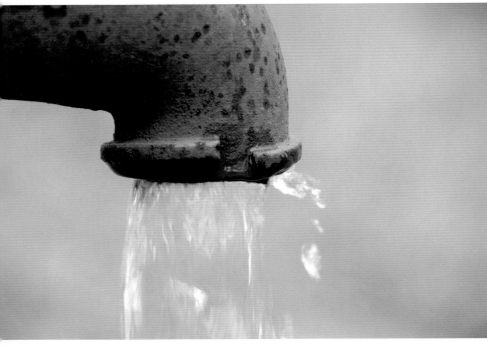
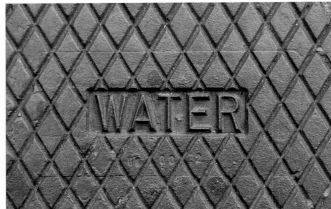
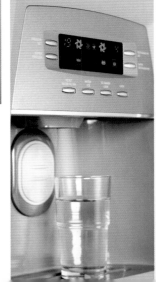
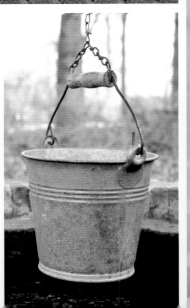

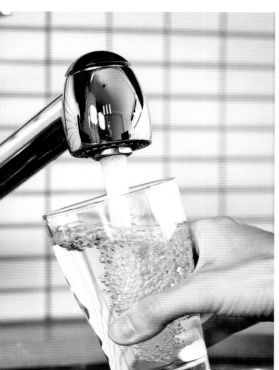
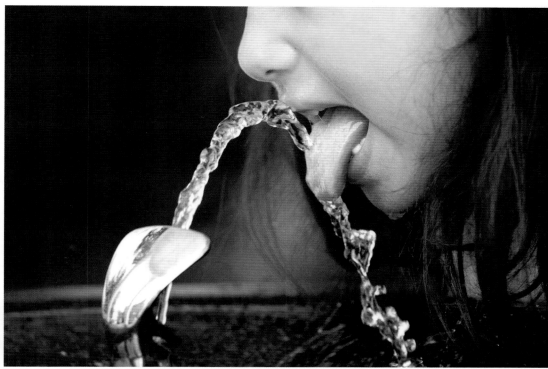
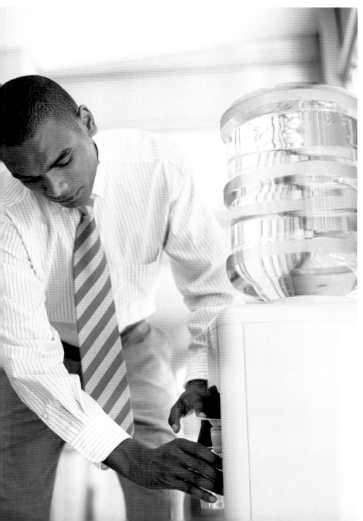
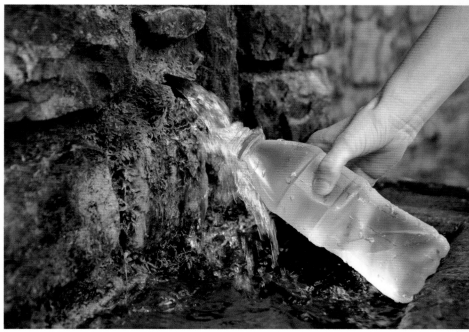

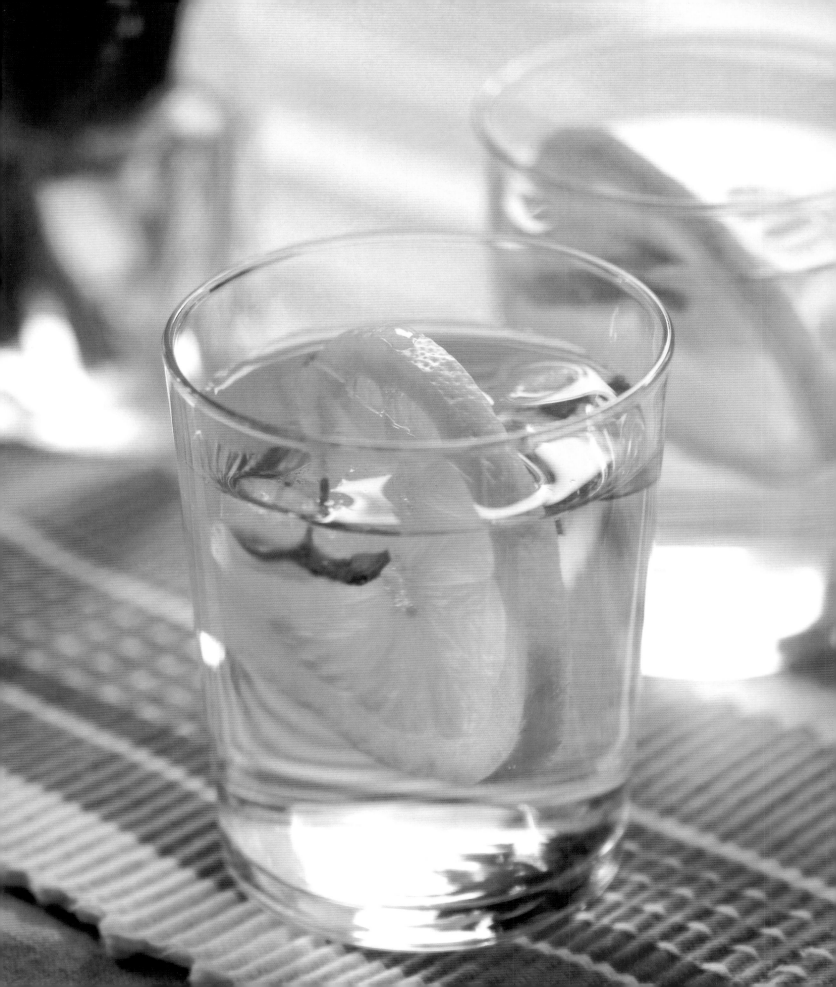

WHAT IF WATER INTAKE IS INADEQUATE?

When we don't provide our bodies with enough water, they attempt to avoid dehydration by decreasing sweat and urine output. If this compensatory mechanism proves inadequate and insufficient fluid intake persists, dehydration will occur. Dehydration causes an impairment of the body cooling mechanisms, along with a possible rise in body temperature and an inefficient clearance of body waste. The blood thickens and blood flow becomes impaired, increasing the risk of intravascular clotting. This may manifest as stroke or heart attack.

Insufficient water intake also leads to constipation—to the delight of the laxative industry.[4] Exercise and fiber intake play a role, as well.

Dehydration may cause a person to experience dizziness or headache. During prolonged, arduous exercise serious dehydration may occur, so careful attention to fluid intake is particularly important under these circumstances. Drinking an inadequate amount of water also increases the risk of developing kidney and gallstones.[5]

In 1995, *The Journal of the American Medical Association* called attention to the hazards facing older Americans from inadequate fluid intake.[6] It's estimated that adequate hydration of older people could save thousands of days of hospitalization and millions of dollars each year. Such an observation has implications for all age groups worldwide.

HOW MUCH WATER IS NEEDED TO STAY HYDRATED?

To help stay hydrated during prolonged physical activity or in hot weather, the 2005 Dietary Guidelines for Americans recommends that we drink fluids during the activity as well as several glasses of water or other fluid after the physical activity is completed.[7]

In the healthy person, a practical guide to water intake is to consume sufficient amounts throughout the day to ensure that the urine is a pale color. (Urine may be a bright yellow color after taking certain medications, including vitamin pills and antituberculosis medication.)

Begin drinking water in the morning, because the body is relatively dehydrated from insensible (invisible) water loss, or perspiration, during sleep. Then continue to drink water at regular intervals throughout the day.

Be sure to drink water that is pure and clean. It is the most healthfully beneficial liquid we can consume because it's relatively free of electrolytes and diuretic agents such as caffeine. Alcoholic drinks, apart from their other deleterious effects, are also diuretic agents. Most soft drinks are loaded with sugar, contributing to problems of obesity, diabetes, and dental caries.

Water cleanses, refreshes, and powerfully aids the body's restoration.

WATER AS A CLEANSING AGENT

Another important use of water is cleansing. Regular bathing removes accumulated dirt and contaminating debris, reducing the risk of infection.

Frequent hand washing may reduce transmission of many infectious agents from person to person. If people thoroughly washed their hands with soap and water before eating and after activities that soil their hands, a large percentage of infectious diseases would be eliminated.

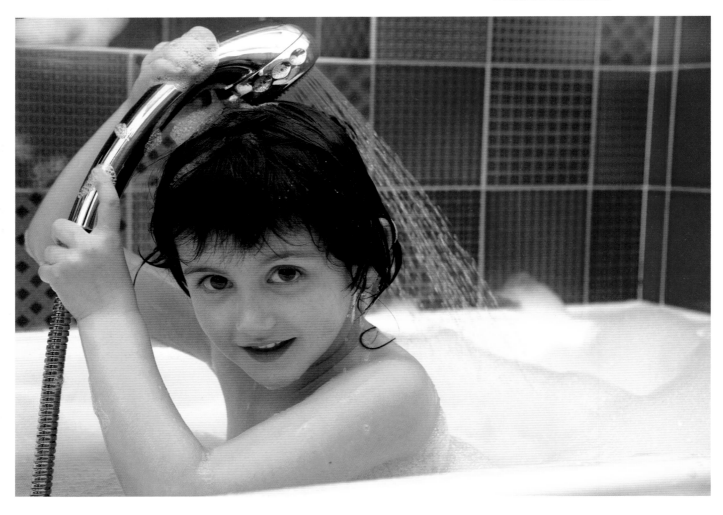

HYDROTHERAPY

Hydrotherapy is the use of water as a simple home therapeutic application. It's best applied as a help for simple muscular aches, pains, and bruises. When dealing with muscular aches, apply hot, wet towels alternated with cold, wet towels (ending with a cold application) to affected areas to improve blood flow. If a recent injury and bruising have occurred, cold compresses are more appropriate. Caution should be exercised where the skin is diseased or cut. When blood flow becomes impaired or there is neurological damage resulting in an inability to feel heat, hot applications may lead to serious injury, so caution is again advised. This is especially applicable to people with diabetes or those whose nerves have been damaged by injury or surgery.

There are many modes of hydrotherapy, such as cold mitten friction, hot foot baths, heat compresses, and ice compresses. It's unfortunate that so few utilize this most useful tool for relief.

A man injured his elbow during a badminton game. He would not listen to advice to compress the hematoma of his elbow with ice, which would reduce the bleeding. The next day the bruised area around his elbow had swollen so much that he went to see the doctor right away. The doctor advised the use of ice compresses at home, and charged a $100 consultation fee!

"The external application of water is one of the easiest and most satisfactory ways of regulating the circulation of the blood. . . . But many have never learned by experience the beneficial effects of the proper use of water. . . . All should become intelligent in its use in simple home treatments."[8]

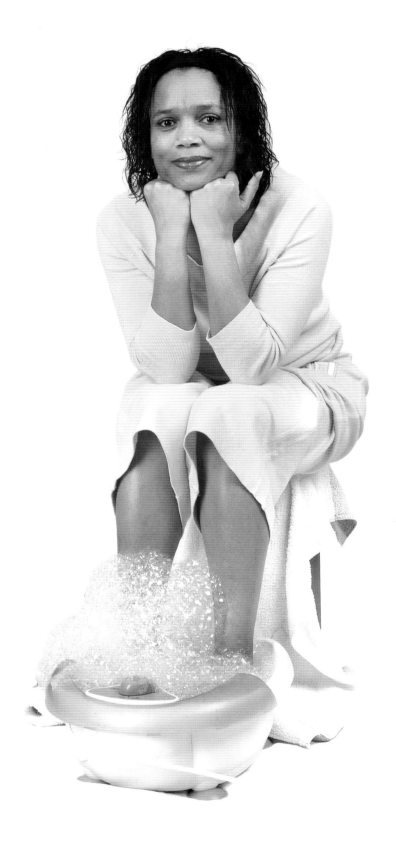

APPROPRIATE CONCERN FOR EARTH'S INHABITANTS

Water is a precious and indispensable resource. It's therefore important to conserve water resources:

1. Avoid wasting water. When possible, install toilets and shower heads in your home that use less water. When brushing your teeth, turn on the water taps only to wet and then rinse your toothbrush; turn taps off while brushing your teeth. Repair leaking faucets; continuous small drips over time can turn into huge amounts of wasted water. Also watch for other appropriate ways to conserve water in your day-to-day routines.

2. Avoid polluting water. Water can be polluted by human excrement, industrial waste, and chemicals. Animals raised in large agricultural feed-lot operations consume huge quantities of water, and their excrement has the potential to pollute groundwater and nearby rivers and streams. Eating a vegetarian diet helps to conserve water, because foods consumed in a plant-based diet require much less water to produce.

WATER OF LIFE

Life cannot exist without water. All body functions require it. Water cleanses, refreshes, and powerfully aids the body's restoration. Similarly, in our spiritual lives, we cannot live eternally without the Water of Life.

What does the term "Water of Life" mean? Two thousand years ago Jesus Christ met a woman in Samaria who had come to a well to draw water. He asked her for a drink, and in the ensuing conversation He said He could give her water that would take away her thirst forever. "'Whoever drinks of this water [from the well] will thirst again,'" Jesus told her, "'but whoever drinks of the water that I shall give him will never thirst. But the water that I shall give him will become in him a fountain of water springing up into everlasting life'" (John 4:13, 14, NKJV). Such a concept implies a spiritual thirst-quenching that would satisfy the yearning for peace, joy, freedom from guilt, forgiveness, and a sense of oneness with God.

Christians find such a solution in the person of Jesus Christ. His life was in marked contrast to the turmoil, strife, jealousy, anger, and dissatisfaction among the people both of His day and ours. His offer to all is that we come to Him and dedicate ourselves to His service. He promises that this will bring relief from toil, anxiety, and stress, providing rest and fulfillment in Him. His offer is still valid today. May we be transformed as we drink, bathe, and are soaked in His compassion, love, and acceptance.

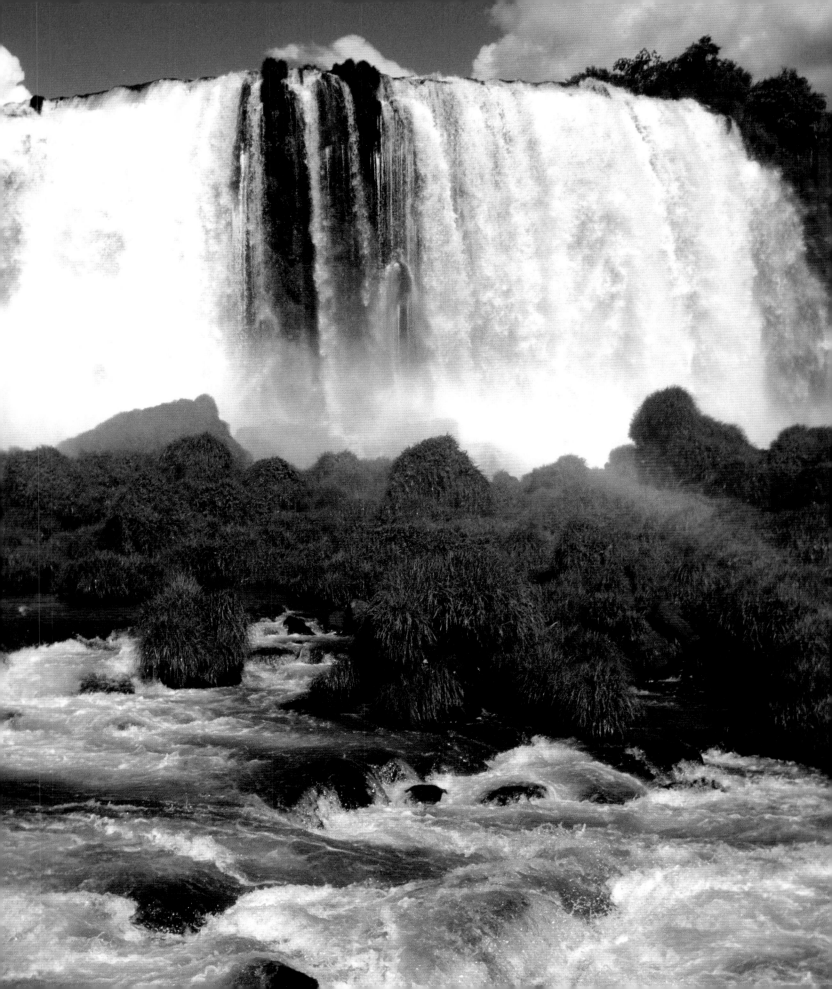

Celebrating Liquids: Life-Application Questions

Take the time to consider these questions and apply what you are learning to your life.

1 Based on my level of activity, how much water does my body lose daily? How much liquid am I taking in every day? Based on the suggested criteria of the color of my urine, am I getting sufficient liquids on a daily basis? What can I do to increase my intake of liquids? Do I need to fill a water bottle each morning and make sure I drink it all? Would a schedule to drink at specific times each day be useful (not forgetting the important first glass in the morning)?

2 What percentage of my liquid intake is pure water? What drinks increase the chance of dehydration because they are diuretic in nature? Do I consume too many sugary drinks (including fruit juices) that contribute to a weight problem? Do I make too many of these drinks readily available for my family, rather than keeping them for special times only?

3 Because a third of the water my body gets comes from my food, do I need to reevaluate the amount of high-water foods I'm eating? Which of the fruits and vegetables mentioned that are high in water content am I going to choose to use more regularly?

4 How often do I use water as a cleansing or healing agent? How should I tactfully remind others to wash their hands more frequently in order to stop the spread of infections? When is it appropriate to use hydrotherapy? Do I have ice or ice packs in my refrigerator for use on bumps or bruises?

GROUP DISCUSSION

5 Ron and his family enjoy exercising outdoors. When it is hot and humid, they drink a lot of sodas to keep hydrated. Sometimes they complain of headaches and dizziness. What is wrong? How could they be encouraged to exercise but also kept safe? What are the symptoms of dehydration and heat stroke?

6 How often do we think about and thank God for the wonderful gift of sufficient water? Which of the suggested ways to conserve water should we begin implementing? Which plant-based foods consume less water in production and reduce the amount of contamination of water supplies?

7 Being thirsty reminds us of the greater thirst for the "water of life" that Jesus offers. How can we accept that gift so that we can also be a source of life to those with whom we interact on a daily basis?

Would a schedule to drink at specific times each day be useful?

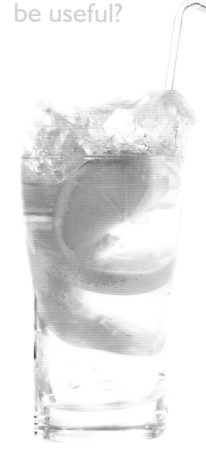

Celebrating the Environment

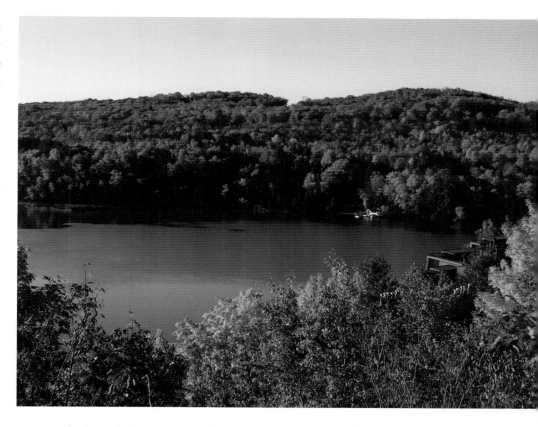

Several years ago my wife, Janet, and I began searching for a country cabin to purchase for weekend retreats. North of Toronto in the Muskoka District we found some beautiful turquoise lakes. We were deeply impressed and admired their tropical colors, only to be told that the lakes were "dead." Acid rain, caused by industrial pollution of the atmosphere, had acidified the water to such a degree that the lakes were devoid of flora and fauna. Beautiful to look at but toxic for any kind of life within them, such lakes have become sterile.

Life can flourish only in a suitable environment; it requires an appropriate balance of climate, water, soil, and air.

The physical, chemical, and biotic factors that surround us, such as air, temperature, sun, soil, and water—as well as the flora and fauna—compose our "environment." Health requires a sustaining and supportive environment, and many of our practices undermine this support and sustainability.

Pollution of water and air, destruction of natural habitats, and massive industrialization threaten the continuation of life as we know it; therefore,

Health requires a sustaining and supportive environment.

environmental awareness is important to the maintenance of health.

Fifty years ago lead poisoning was relatively common. Physicians were taught to recognize discoloration of gums, bluish stippling in blood cells, and the sight of neurotoxic damage caused by lead. Lead was added to paint to give it luster and strength, but children would pick at flaking paint, eat the flakes, and become poisoned by the lead content. Gasoline contained lead to augment its properties with resultant increased atmospheric lead that could be inhaled and therefore poison the populace. Recognition of the cause of a problem often leads to a resolution, as in the now ubiquitous production of lead-free gasoline.

OVERPOPULATION: AN ENVIRONMENTAL CONCERN?

A little pollution here, destruction of a few trees there, the dumping of some raw sewage into a river somewhere—all these may seem of small impact. When such isolated acts are multiplied by millions, however, they begin to have a major destructive effect. It's for this reason that many people are beginning to voice what has sometimes been labeled a "politi- cally incorrect" viewpoint: that overpopulation is the worst environmental threat we are faced with today.

A single automobile may emit what would be insignificant pollutants if it were the only vehicle in the world; but as the world's population burgeons, the number of automobiles rockets, too.

Current projections—incorporating projected declines in growth rates—still predict a global population somewhere between 8 and 10.5 billion by the year 2050.[1] The effects of overpopulation depend on the ratio of population to sustainable resources, as well as on the distribution of such resources, including clean water, clean air, food, shelter, and appropriate climatic conditions.

Overpopulation often damages a nation's economy. When a country is unable to feed its population, it consequently has to purchase and import food. People take up space needed for farms and forests; their waste pollutes the water, land, and air. Destruction of forests results in loss of animal habitats as well as loss of plant species and their capacity to remove carbon dioxide and produce oxygen. Overpopulation presents serious difficulties to effective governance and stress; consequently, strife and turmoil often ensue.

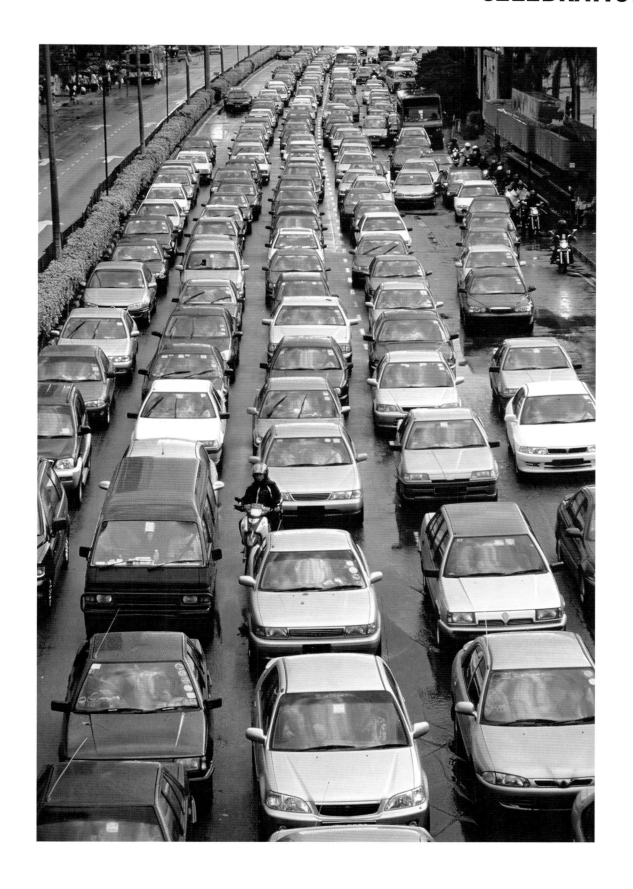

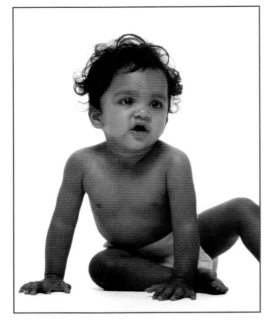
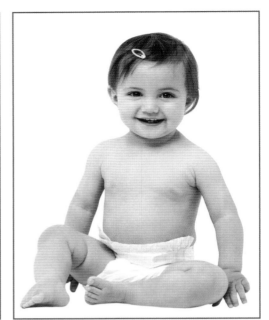
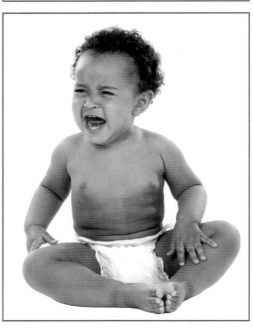
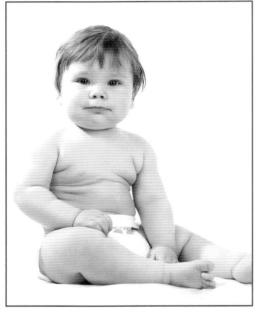
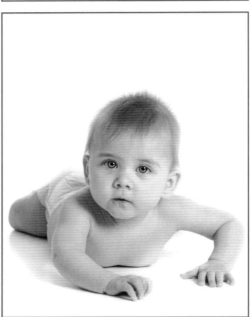
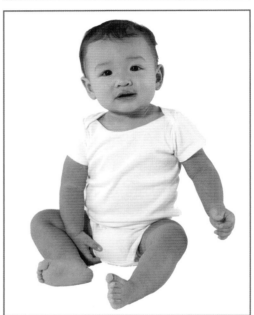
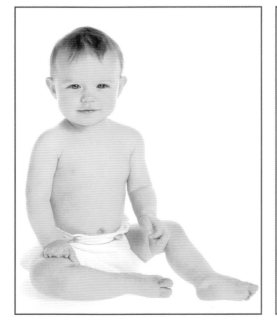
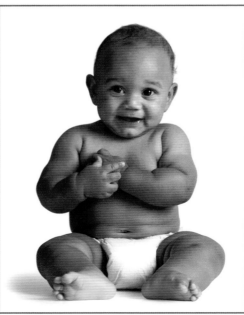
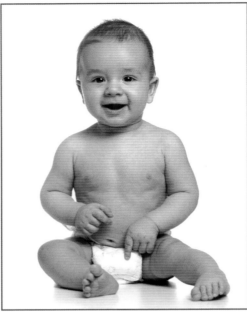

Between 1950 and 2005, the number of children born per woman decreased from 5.02 to 2.65, though even at this rate the global population continues to expand. By continent, the numbers (for 1950 to 2005) are seen in the table below:[2]

Continent/Region	Numbers
Europe	2.66 to 1.41
North America	3.47 to 1.99
Oceania	3.87 to 2.30
Central America	6.38 to 2.66
South America	5.75 to 2.49
Asia	5.85 to 2.43
Middle East and North Africa	6.99 to 3.37
Sub-Saharan Africa	6.70 to 5.53

Many people are beginning to voice what has sometimes been labeled a "politically incorrect" viewpoint: that overpopulation is the worst environmental threat we are faced with today.

SUSTAINABLE AGRICULTURE

Closely related to overpopulation is the issue of sustainable agriculture. Improvements in agricultural technology have led to enormous increases in yields of produce per acre of land utilized. Such improvements, however, do not come without an environmental cost. Further changes in agricultural priorities are needed to balance the utilization of land.

DEFORESTATION

Deforestation on a massive scale often results in damage to the quality of the land. Although some 30 percent of the earth's surface is still covered by forest, large tracts of land are lost annually to deforestation.

FOOD DISTRIBUTION

The balance between our need for forests and our need for food relates to the pressures of overpopulation. Deforestation contributes to climate change. Moist forest soils quickly dry out without the shade of a forest canopy. Forest lands can quickly become deserts. The role played by forests in absorbing greenhouse gases is a central one.[3]

The uneven development of the world means that although current food production is sufficient for the global population, food is not freely available to all. Poverty and the impact of climate change are felt much more acutely where drought and desertification are taking place. Many undeveloped countries have an inadequate infrastructure to permit the proper distribution of food.

CLIMATE CHANGE

Most scientists agree that there have been significant warming changes during the last 100 years, though opinions differ as to why.

Climate change may influence food production. Yields of grain have been shown in many situations to vary with temperatures. For example, the International Rice Research Institute in the Philippines[4] found that rice production declined by 10 percent for each 1-degree-centigrade increase in growing season nighttime-minimum temperature.

Researchers Lobell and Field[5] reported that climate changes since 1981 have resulted in annual losses of wheat, maize, and barley, representing roughly a combined loss of $5 billion per year as of 2002. This is not a sizable amount, however, relative to the value of improved yields resulting from technological change.

ENERGY CONSERVATION

Reliance upon fossil fuels has characterized much of the energy utilization during the past century. It's likely that the increased cost of such energy will drive the move to alternate energy

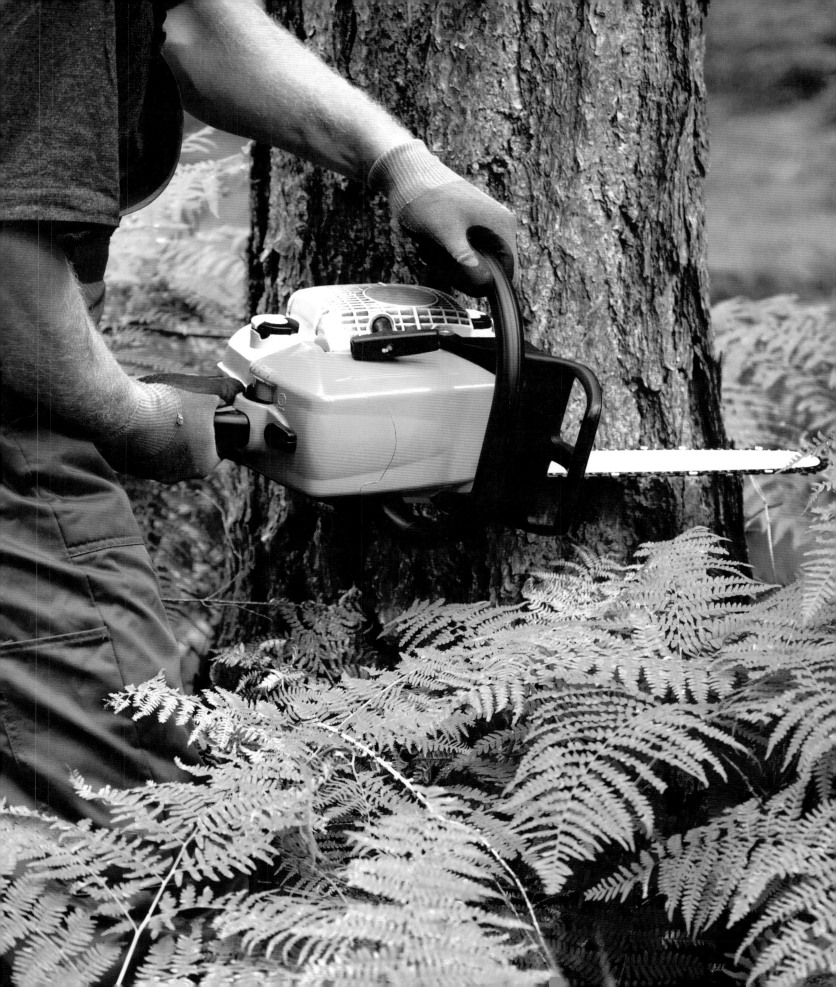

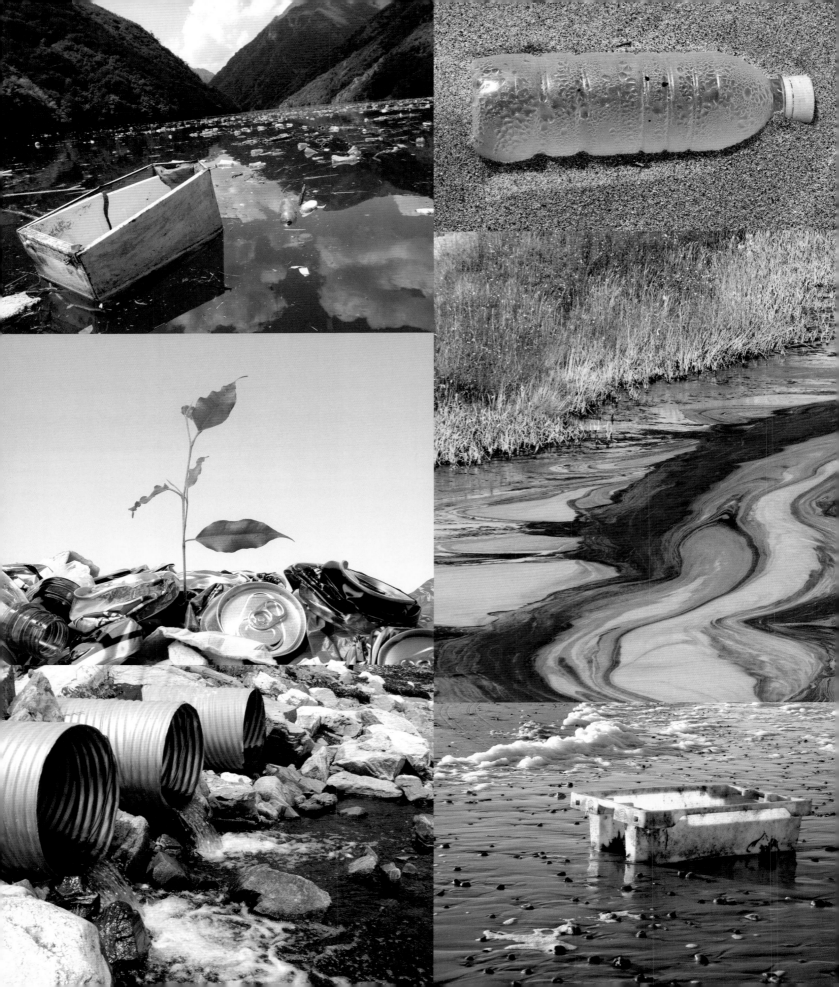

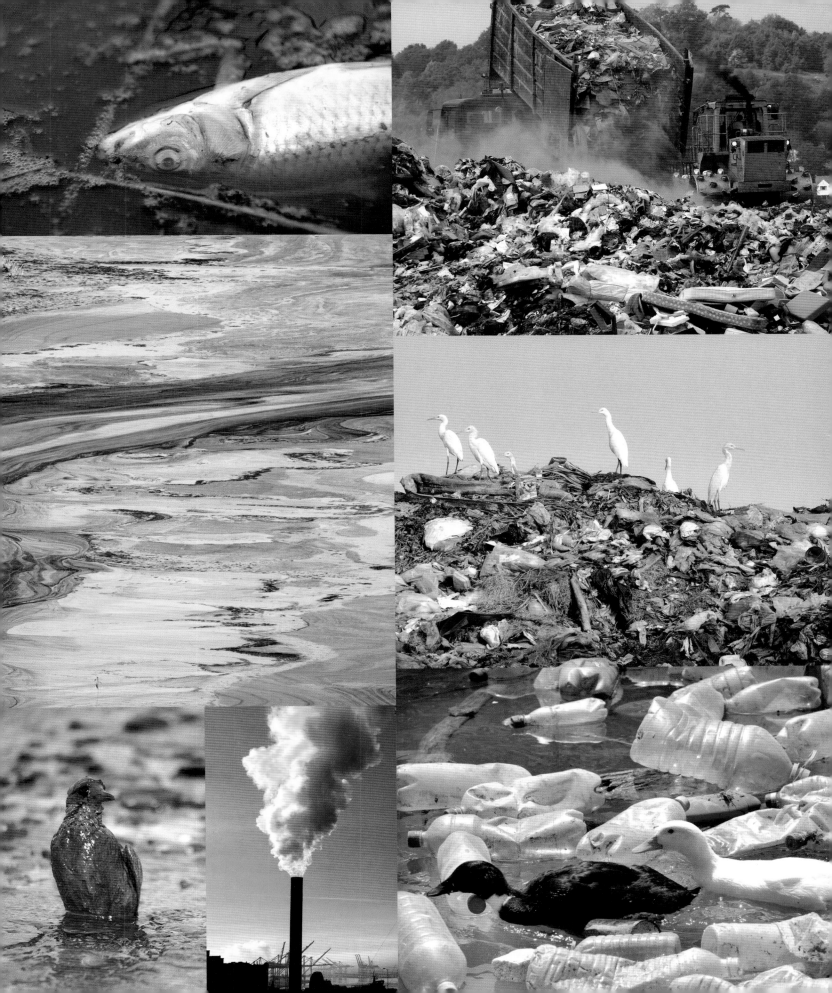

sources. Regardless of cost issues, energy conservation is an important part of environment preservation.

POLLUTION

Two areas of pollution that are particularly concerning are water and air pollution.

Industrialization has produced massive amounts of collateral waste material. The seriousness of environment contamination by pollutants varies with the elements involved. Plastics are derivatives of petroleum-type products, and while extremely useful, they do not naturally degrade easily. It's been shown that plastic can persist for multiple decades. Even when mixed with cellulose to produce so-called "biodegradable plastic," the actual plastic particles remain much longer than the cellulose, which degrades. Remaining plastic particles, if small enough, may be subject to bacterial degradation. In practice, such degradation does not always occur as predicted. The state of California sued a plastic bottle maker—ENSO Plastics, Aquamantra and Balance Water—for false claims.[6]

Sun, wind, and wave action merely fragment plastic, but eventually most of it finds its way into the ocean. Scientists have discovered plastic particulate matter at a depth of 15 to 30 feet in the Pacific Ocean. These particles, called "nurdles," have been found in the digestive tracts of krill, which are the ocean's basic food source for most marine life. Our addiction to disposable plastic water bottles may pose a huge threat to the planet.[7]

Industrial waste—which includes heavy metals such as lead, mercury, and cadmium, as well as the toxic dioxin compounds—can be particularly dangerous and is contaminating the underground water. The radioactive contamination following the 2011 earthquake and massive tsunami off the coast of Japan will likely render the Fukushima area uninhabitable for decades, if not centuries. The Chernobyl disaster in Ukraine in 1986 resulted in increases in thyroid and other cancers. Radioactive isotopes leached into the water are a form of silent yet lethal pollution.

DOMESTIC AND AGRICULTURAL WASTE

Outbreaks of disease frequently are related to viral and bacterial contamination by human and animal waste. Hygiene is a fundamental health principle.

The Blacksmith Institutes Technical Advisory Board[8] reports that persons living in polluted regions may not have immediate health problems, but may later develop cancers, lung infections, and mental retardation.

There are towns in various parts of the world where life expectancy currently approaches low medieval rates, and where birth defects are the norm rather than the exception. In other places, children's asthma rates have been measured above 90 percent. In these re-

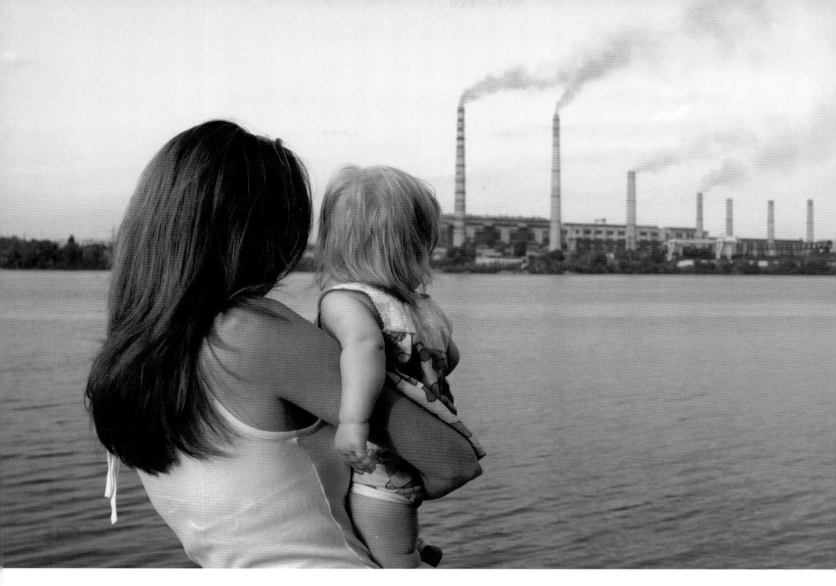

gions, life expectancy may be half that of the richest nations. In North America, it's estimated that half the population is affected by some form of dangerous pollution levels.

The American Lung Association[9] estimates that roughly 50 percent of Americans live in counties that have unhealthful levels of either ozone or pesticide pollution. The University of Southern California[10] has studied residents in 12 communities within a 200-mile radius of Los Angeles. They have followed three groups of children within these communities and quite convincingly have shown interference with lung growth in those who live in more polluted atmospheric conditions. Such children are at increased risk of bronchial and pulmonary disease. Follow-up studies have confirmed these findings.

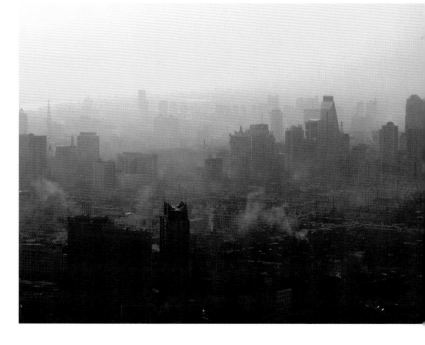

SOLAR IRRADIATION

The sun is central to the provision of energy to our planet. Much of its radiation is important to well-being, but overexposure to ultraviolet radiation can be harmful. Such radiation may be stronger should the ozone layers of the upper atmosphere be depleted.

Sunshine maintains the ambient temperature of the earth; it promotes photosynthesis, which is the fundamental food-producing mechanism. Sunlight powers the recycling of water through evaporation of water into the clouds, and its distillation as rain.

Sunshine also converts an inactive form of vitamin D called cholecalciferol into the active form of vitamin D we need for so many bodily functions. While some of us live in situations of adequate sunlight, many of us work indoors and do not get sufficient exposure to the sun. Darkly pigmented skin does not permit the effect of sunlight to the same extent as pale skin, so vitamin D levels may be lower in such people, especially when they live in extreme northern or southern climes.

Dermatologists have noted the association between sunburn and skin cancer, and advocate the avoidance of overexposure. An appropriate amount depends on the pigmentation of our skin, our geographic location, and the season.

On the other hand, vitamin D is probably an important factor in controlling the growth of other cancers, such as prostate cancer. Sunlight exposure, therefore, in an appropriate amount, is essential to health.[11] It kills many bacteria, and it's a healthful practice to let the sunlight stream into our homes.

Sunlight also stimulates the production of serotonin. This is an example of the "external" environment influencing our "internal" environment. The Seasonal Affective Disorder (SAD) first described in 1984 by Dr. Norman Rosenthal, a neuropsychiatrist

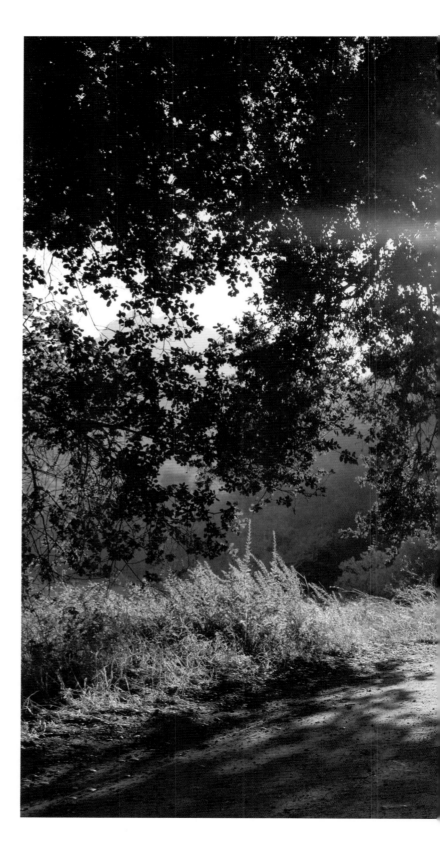

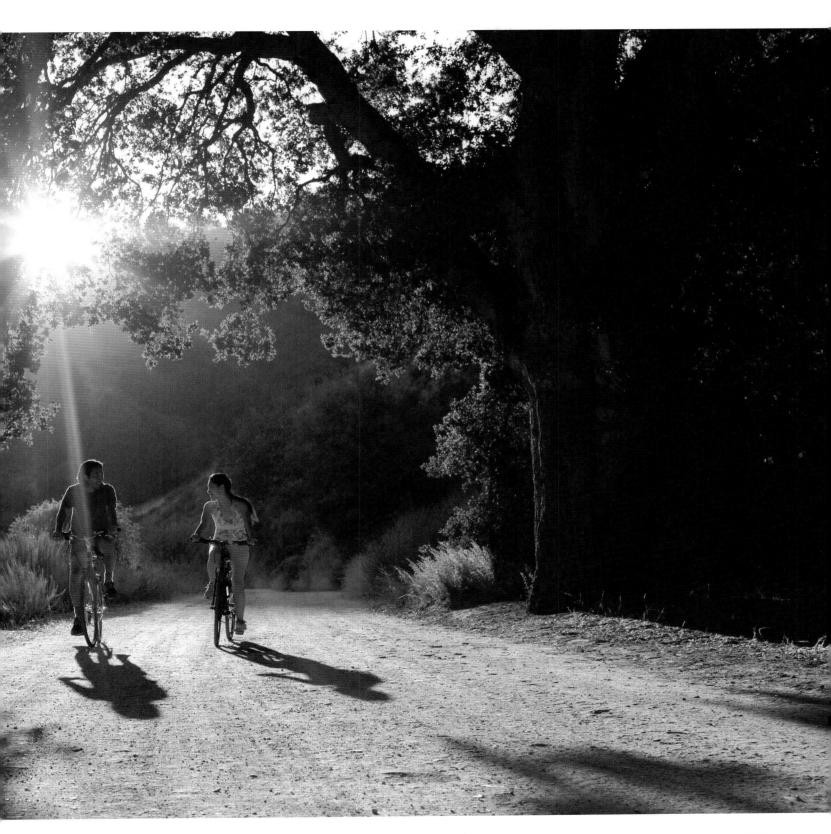

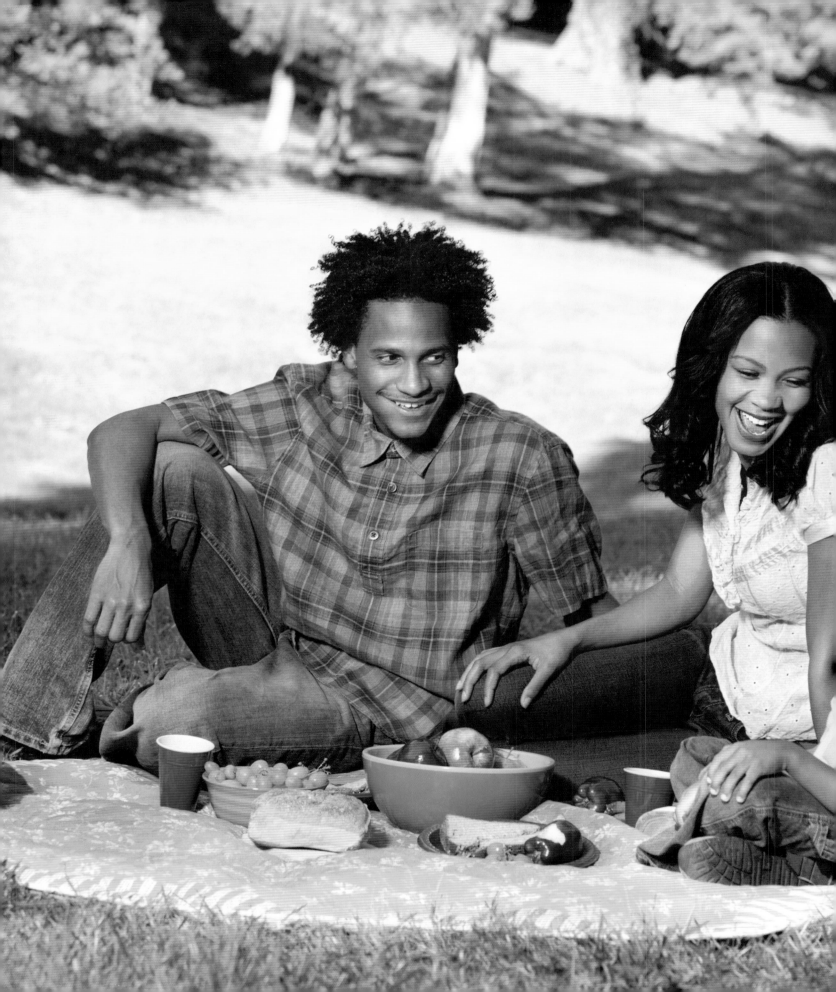

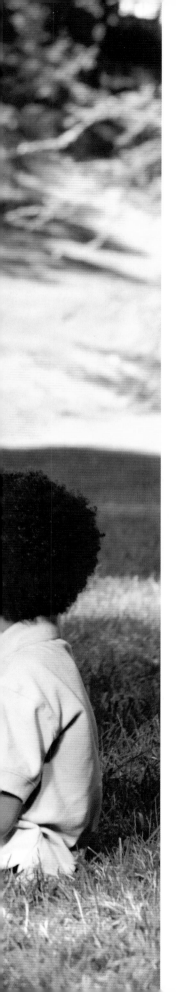

at the National Institute of Mental Health, affects many during the winter months when light is diminished. Such people suffer a loss of energy, alteration in appetite, somnolence (drowsiness), irritability, and depression.[12] They will benefit by exposure to bright light.

INTERNAL ENVIRONMENT

Although we live in an external environment, our metabolic processes take place in an internal environment.

Our bodies maintain a precise balance—or equilibrium—through the processes of homeostasis. We best support homeostasis by a life that includes daily physical activity and a healthful diet rich in unrefined plant foods.

We must be extremely careful not to introduce toxins of overt and dangerous action into our bodies' internal environment. Tobacco smoke, with its hundreds of chemicals, is a prime example. Alcohol also is a potent toxin. The use of psychotropic drugs (medications that affect the central nervous system and can cause changes in behavior or perception) as "recreational" substances intoxicates our internal environment, as well.

Many substances have never been tested or properly evaluated, yet are touted as being good for one or another condition. Without evidence, we use them in a vacuum of knowledge. Many so-called "natural" substances of herbal or plant origin fall into such categories and are best avoided.

HOME ENVIRONMENT

Health, God's gift to us, is best maintained in the most natural state of unpolluted and hygienic purity. We are stewards of the earth, responsible for managing the earth's resources and the environment of our bodies.

Because we are more than mere physical beings and possess intellectual, emotional, and spiritual dimensions, we also need to consider the emotional and spiritual environments in which we live. Too many homes are places of tension and distrust. Anger and violence in the home will take an enormous toll on the health of our children and ourselves.

Domestic violence affects many of our homes; verbal abuse also is common. Our homes should provide an oasis of security in a world of turmoil. Kind and supportive attitudes will nurture the emotional health of the family.

The spiritual environment of the home affects the environment of our minds. Our homes should be calm, comforting, and supportive places. Values are taught and come from a basis of belief and trust. We place our trust in a loving God. We are secure in His care and teach our children to seek this spiritual relationship with Him. We urge them to be loving and nonjudgmental of others. God admonishes us to love our enemies, and to do good to those who might mistreat us.[13]

If we live in an atmosphere of tolerance and peace, our spiritual environment will also be conducive to health. We will, as it were, drink at a fountain of life. The atmosphere of heaven will comfort our souls. We will be secure as we ground ourselves in the certainty of God's love.

Celebrating the Environment: Life-Application Questions

Take the time to consider these questions and apply what you are learning to your life.

1 Have I experienced any of the Seasonal Affective Disorder (SAD) symptoms, such as depression and irritability, in the winter months or when spending time indoors? How can I change my program in order to spend a carefully regulated amount of time in the sunshine? Are there children in my community or family who need encouragement to spend time outdoors, or who need caution to limit their exposure to too much sunshine?

2 Which pollutants is my body being exposed to? Which of these can I limit or eliminate altogether? Are some of my choices exposing me to chemicals or substances that might give me passing gratification but have harmful effects in the long-term?

3 How am I contributing emotionally and spiritually to the following environments: home, work, school, church, community? What type of contribution am I making? Is it causing pollution or peace, strife or sanctuary? What choices can I make, and where can I receive the help I need to stick to my decision, to improve and protect my environment?

GROUP DISCUSSION

4 Even though we sometimes may feel as though one person cannot do much to stop deforestation and industrial pollution, besides financially supporting some environmental groups, what choices can we make, such as the ways we use energy and plastics, that will contribute even in a small way to protecting the environment?

5 Shawn has a "green" friend who is highly vocal about environmental issues, but she's skeptical of Shawn's choice to be a vegetarian. Which advantages of a vegetarian diet could Shawn point out that would meet with her friend's approval as an environmentalist?

6 Education can often lead to more informed choices about family size population growth and better quality of life and health to all. In what ways can we support the efforts of groups that run educational institutions and programs in countries where poverty drastically reduces the quality of life for many families?

How can I change my program in order to spend a carefully regulated amount of time in the sunshine?

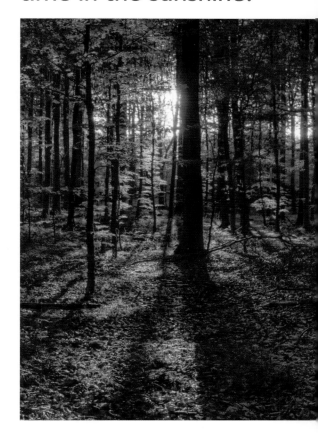

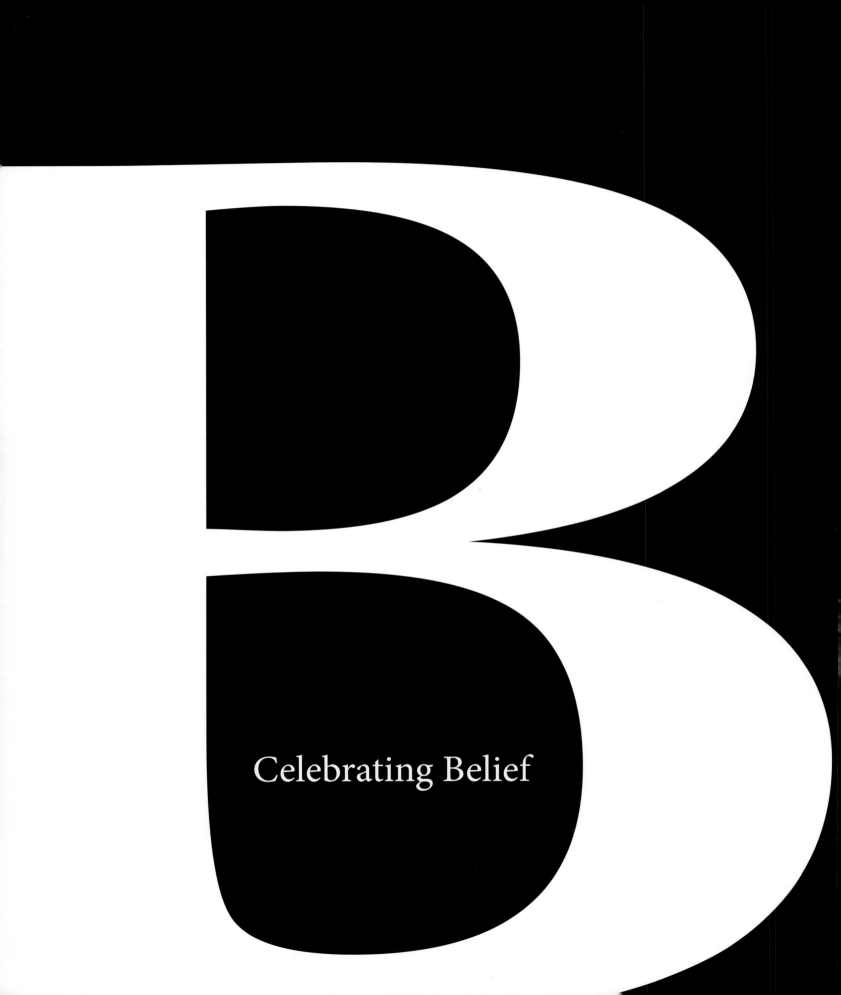

Celebrating Belief

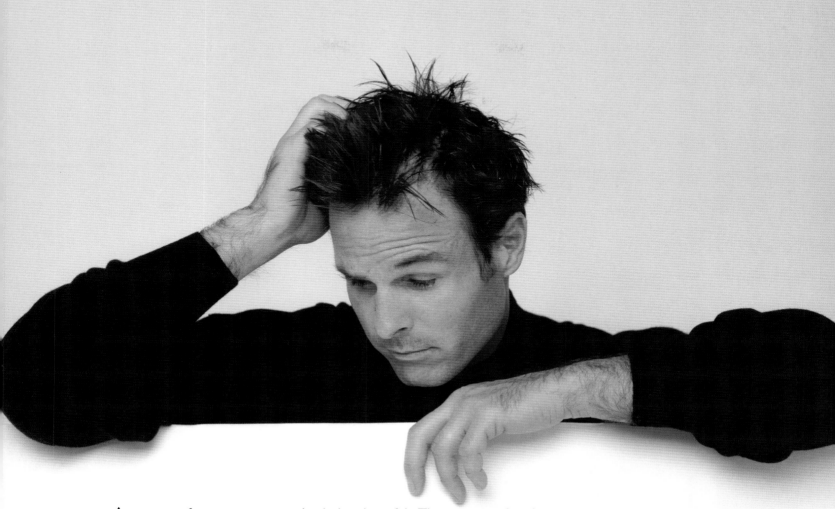

A professor announced to a brand new class of medical students: "I have good news and bad news: The good news is that half of the material you learn in medical school will survive all scrutiny and investigation. It will be enduring. The other half of what we teach you, however, will be proven incorrect. The bad news is we have no way of knowing which half is which!"

In today's world it's sometimes difficult to know what to believe about much of the information we're "fed"! One day we read that drinking alcohol is harmful. The next week other reports indicate that it's protective of good health. Chocolate is fattening, right? Wait a minute—now a research group has reported that it actually helps people lose weight. Coffee is harmful, we've been told. But then we learn that in a significant study those who drank large amounts of coffee lived longer! And one week a major tech company introduces another time-saving, "must have" device; the next week media report those claims as based on unreliable analyses.

In what or whom can we truly believe? Sometimes determining the an-

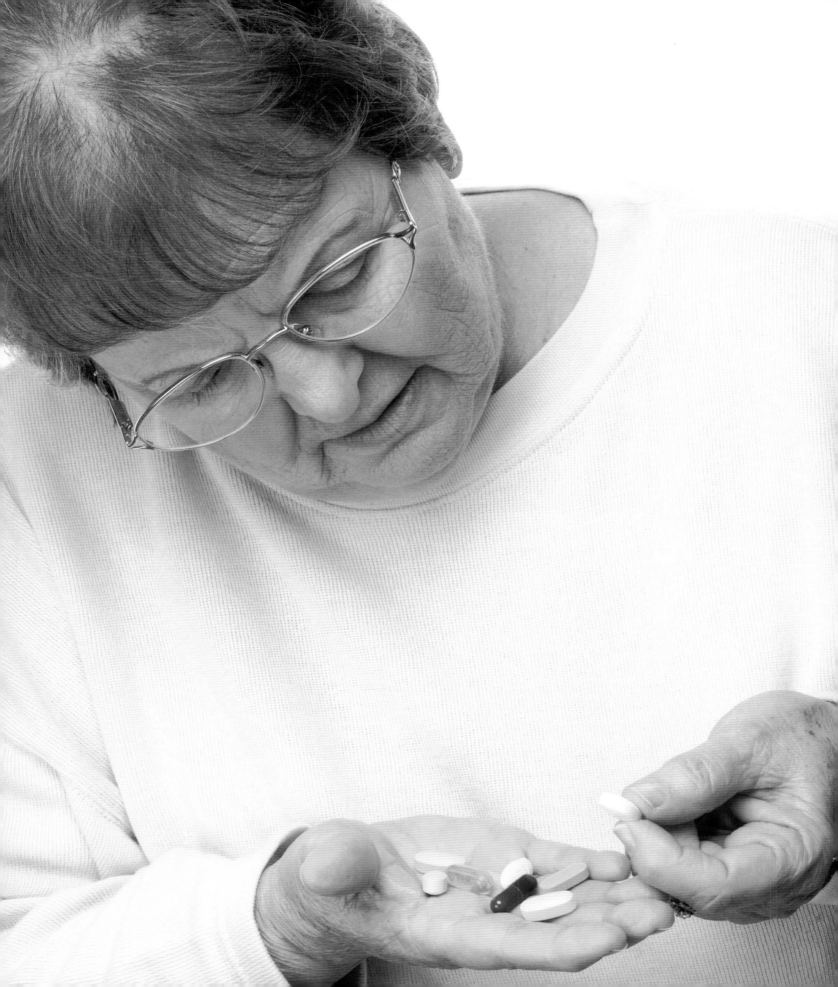

swer to this question is tough! Yet, we all believe in something. The greatest skeptics have beliefs, even if it's the belief that no one can be trusted. The survival of all humans is based on beliefs of some kind. Belief is essential to human existence and organization.

POWER OF BELIEF

One day a physician was examining a patient who complained about a myriad of symptoms, unrelated to any known syndrome or disease complex. The patient told the doctor that perhaps an evil spell had been cast on him and was making him ill. The doctor then took two small glass tubes and filled one with hydrogen peroxide and the other with water. The patient didn't know the two liquids were different. The physician then drew a small amount of blood from the patient and put a few drops into the tube with the hydrogen peroxide. Naturally, there was an immediate reaction of effervescence, and the doctor knowingly nodded. "Ah-ha," he said, "you will benefit from this." He then gave the patient a saline injection and told him to wait in the waiting room.

After a short time the doctor called the patient back into his office and again drew a small amount of blood, this time putting a few drops into the tube containing plain water. As expected, it mixed without any reaction. The doctor told the patient that the evil spell had been broken, and the patient left feeling immensely better. The story goes that the patient told all his friends about how he had been healed, and many of them came to the doctor wanting the same treatment!

As this story demonstrates, there is tremendous power in belief. For many a peddler of "quack medicine," this phenomenon is a mighty source of revenue. "Unscrupulous" salespersons can sometimes create a false need in the minds of their targets. They then sell herbal concoctions, nonessential mineral supplements, nutraceuticals (fortified foods or supplements), special diets, and magnetic or electrical cures mediated through empty black boxes or mild shock-emitting equipment. They are trading on what can be called the "gullibility factor." For those who are healthy, the only cost is some money, from which they are soon parted. In a situation in which something such as cancer is involved, sometimes the delay before undertaking more traditional treatment leads to a deadly outcome as well as the wasting of limited and precious resources on worthless "cure-alls." It's important to place our belief and trust in that which is reliable and not on such unproven methods.

Belief—or faith, within a religious setting—has been shown to have statistically significant benefits that exceed the placebo effect. When the religious experience of Americans who reached the age of 100 was studied, researchers found that religiosity significantly enhanced health. Although many questions are still unanswered, the benefits of trust in God result from more than simply attending religious services.[1]

A study comparing mortality rates between secular and religious kibbutzim (collective agricultural communities in Israel), found a decreased mortality rate over a 15-year follow-up in the religious group. The age-adjusted risk of premature death of members of the secular kibbutz was 1.8 times higher for males and 2.7 times higher for females when compared with the religious kibbutz.[2]

A study of African-Americans found that those who engaged in organized religious activities had improved health and life satisfaction.[3] Duke University research-

er C. G. Ellison found that a lack of religious affiliation increases the risk of depression in African-Americans.[4]

A connection between social relationships and survival has been documented in several studies. C. J. Schoenbach, et al. have documented this effect, particularly among white males.[5]

IMPROVED QUALITY OF LIFE

One of the most consistent findings across all racial groups is that spirituality profoundly improves the quality of life. Ellison describes these significant benefits, brought about by exercising faith:[6]

■ Religious attendance and private devotion strengthen a person's religious belief system.

■ Strong religious systems, when accompanied by a high level of religious certainty, have a substantial and positive influence on well-being.

■ Individuals with strong religious faith report higher levels of life satisfaction, greater personal happiness, and fewer negative psychosocial consequences of traumatic life events.

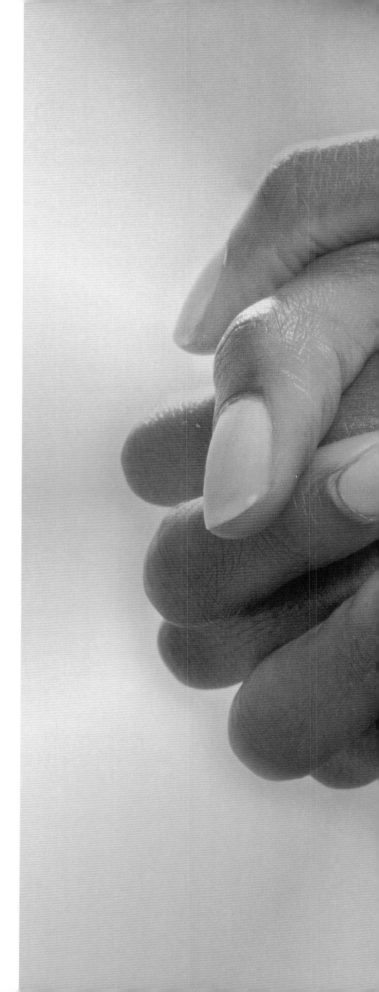

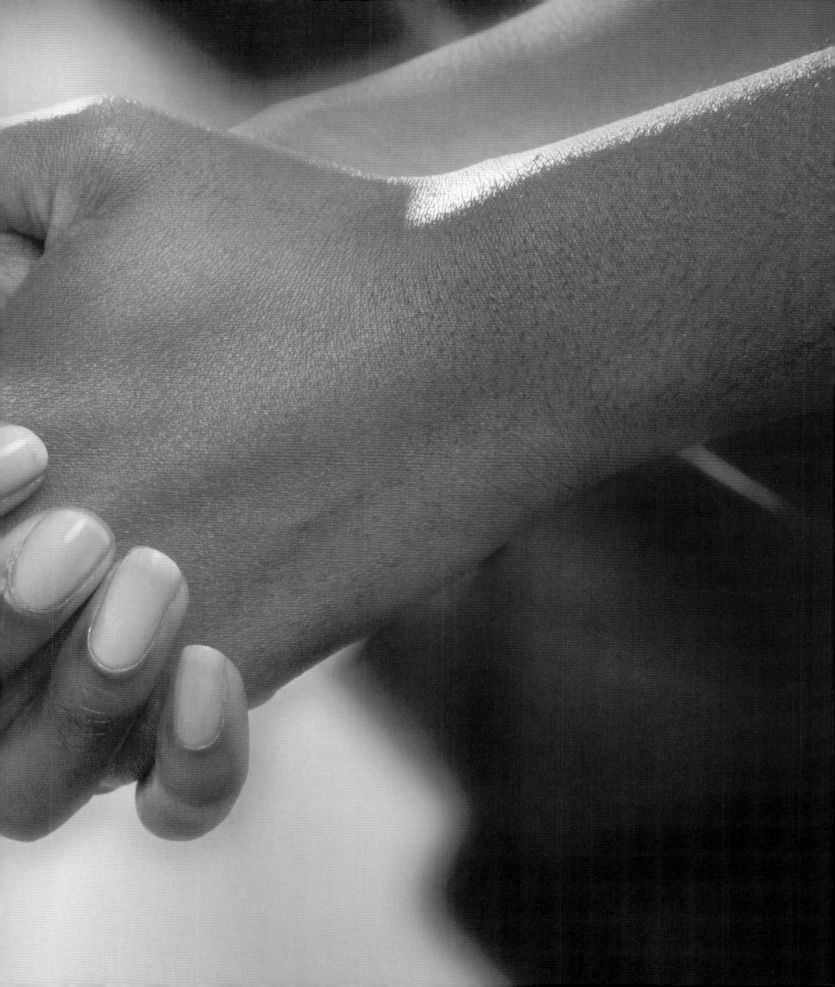

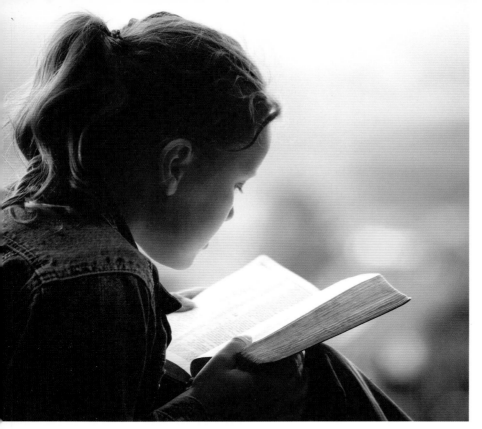
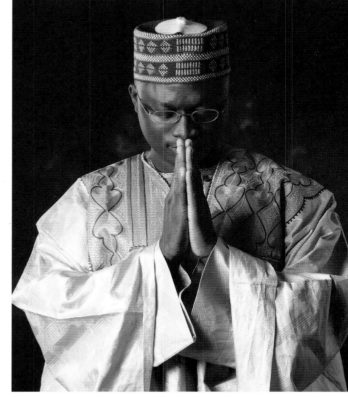
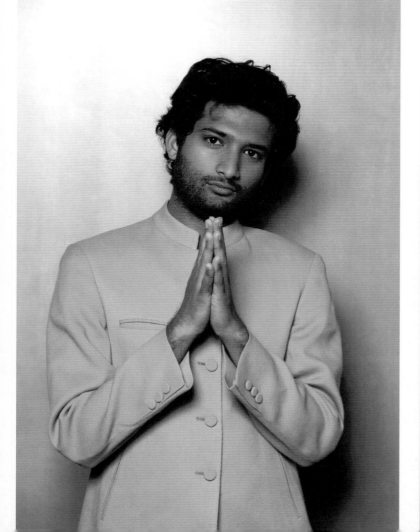
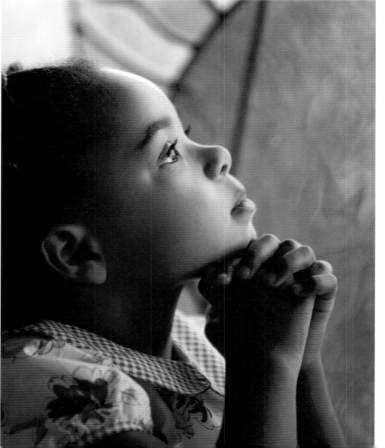

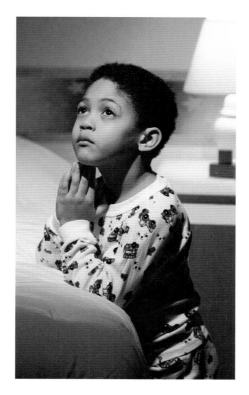

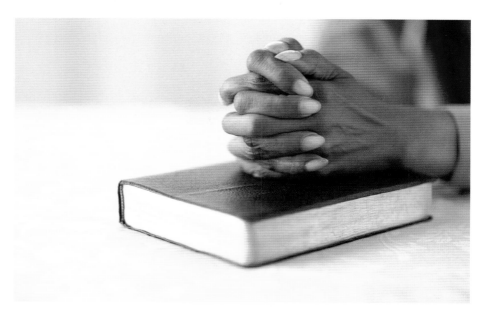

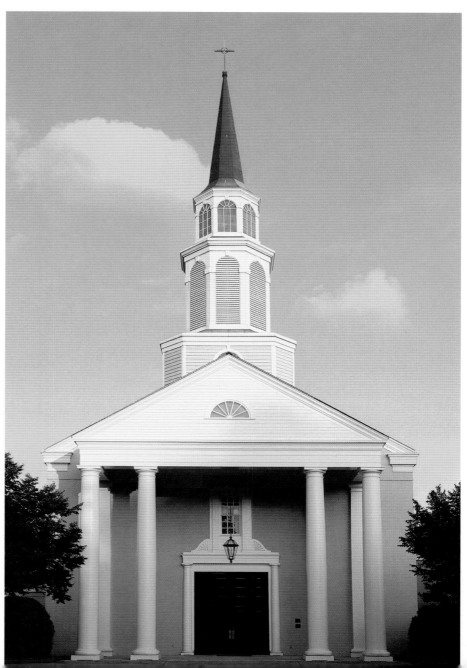

Spirituality not only helps believers but also benefits the nonbelievers in their community. Research has found that communities gain health benefits when they have higher numbers of adherents to faiths that emphasize implicit obedience to God and His standards of conduct.[7] The reason that nonbelievers are benefitted as well is likely that their social norms favor conformity to the more healthful lifestyle embraced by their religious neighbors.

Religious people—particularly adolescents from religious homes who frequently attend religious services, pray, and read Scripture—have fewer problems with alcohol, tobacco, or other drugs than do their nonreligious peers.[8]

Religion was also positively associated with emotionally healthful values and socially accepted behaviors such as tutoring or other volunteer activities often promoted by religious organizations.[9]

The path of those who do what is right is like the first gleam of dawn. It shines brighter and brighter until the full light of day.

Proverbs 4:18, NIRV

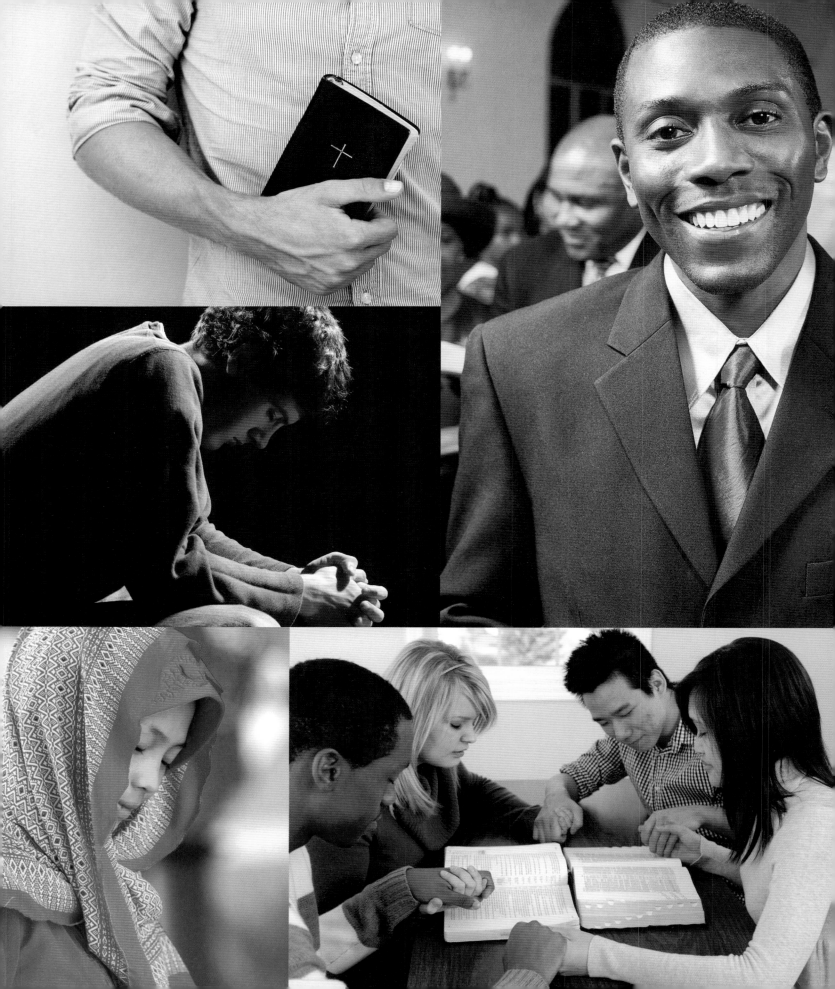

Harold G. Koenig, M.D., discusses the findings of Idler and Kasl. These researchers noted a connection between healthier emotional lives and closer social ties in religiously active people, which often resulted in lower levels of disability. The increased physical activity associated with leisure and social activities did not fully account for the increased benefits in these people's lifestyles, and the authors concluded: "A significant effect of religiousness remains even after social activities have been considered."[10]

Thus, we find that belief in a loving God produces a very positive and powerful health-promoting state of mind. There is nothing more reassuring than the peace and satisfaction experienced by those who place their lives in the hands of a loving God and who are aware of His love for them. This brings health, happiness, and a sense of purpose. As the Bible says, "Those who love your instructions have great peace and do not stumble" (Ps. 119:165, NLT).

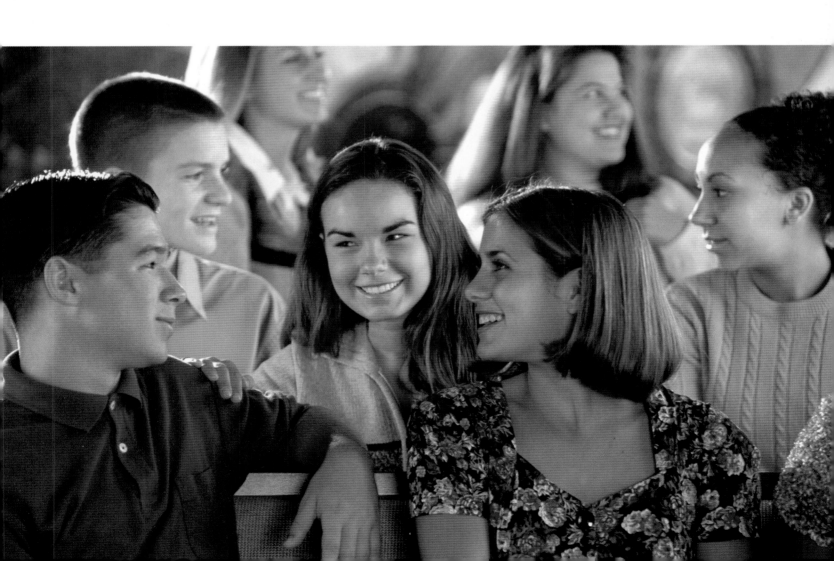

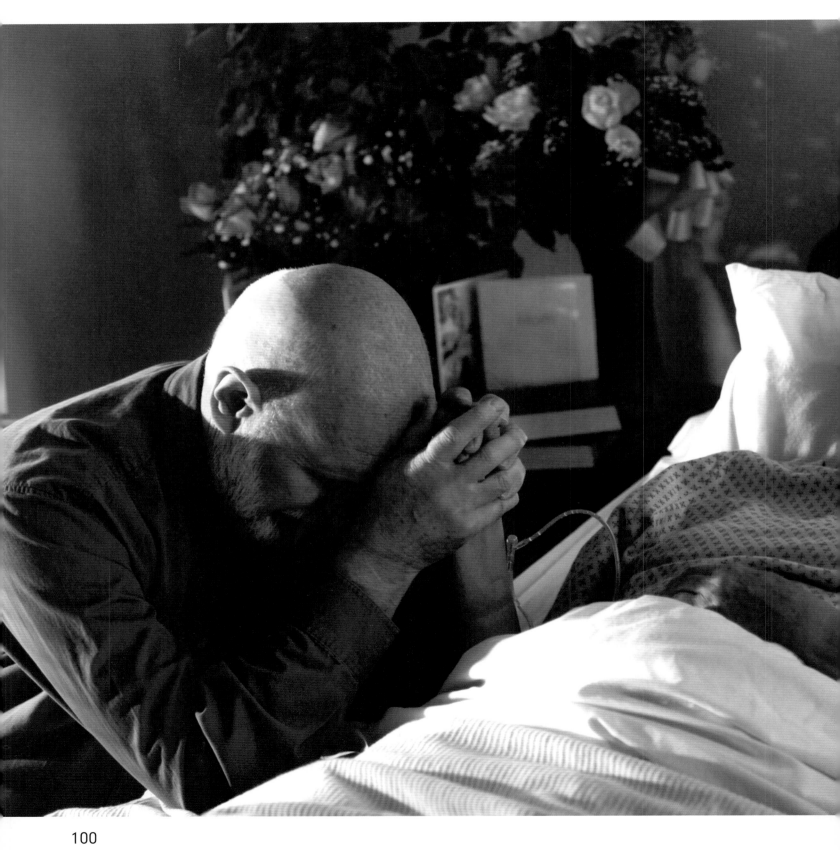

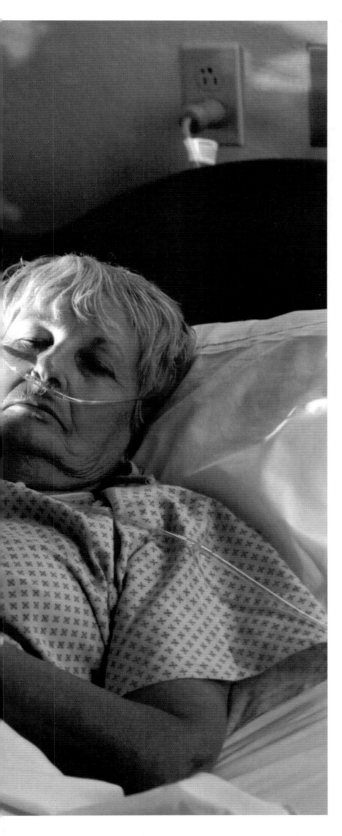

STRESS ISSUES

Belief in God may be associated with reduction in stress, depression, and loneliness. A 1990 Gallup poll revealed that more than 36 percent of Americans live with chronic feelings of loneliness. According to a Princeton University Research Associates survey, at least two thirds of Americans feel stressed at least once a week. Stress, loneliness, and related depression can have serious consequences. Between 75 and 90 percent of all doctor visits contain components relating to stress.[11]

Medical science has discovered that when you feel stressed as a result of facing challenges, the negative emotions trigger the release of certain hormones that stimulate the nervous system in such a way as to put stress on the various organs of the body. If these organs are subjected to stress over long periods of time, they become weakened. Once weakened, they are more susceptible to a variety of disease processes. The order and intensity with which organs are affected depend upon the person's heredity, constitution, environment, and lifestyle. For example:

■ Stress may cause the release of adrenaline, making the heart beat more rapidly and powerfully. Such stress can cause one to suffer from heart palpitations (unpleasant awareness of heartbeat).

■ When stress hormones cause the blood vessels to constrict, they may augment the effects of hypertension and cause diminished peripheral vascular flow, leading to cold hands and feet.

■ Stress may induce shallow and rapid breathing with bronchial dilation, which causes hyperventilation.

■ Stress results in diversion of the blood supply away from the digestive system, possibly affecting digestive processes.

■ Stress induces a state of increased clotting of the blood; though protective in some circumstances, it could have detrimental effects in others.

■ Chronic stressful conditions may increase perspiration, leading to unpleasant dampness.

■ Stress causes an increase in blood glucose (to serve as a rapid source of energy); in those predisposed to diabetes, chronic stress may lead to the hastening of the onset or exacerbation of diabetes mellitus. Stress may cause alterations in gastrointestinal and urinary functions. Some may suffer from urinary frequency and irritable bowel syndrome.

■ A stressed person may visit the doctor for numerous physical complaints and suffer from emotional disorders such as anxiety, depression, phobias, cognitive disorders, memory problems, and sleep disorders.

BENEFITS OF PRAYER

An Ohio study[12] examined the effects of prayer on well-being. Of the 560 respondents, 95 percent classified themselves as religious people; 54 percent were Protestants and 25 percent Catholics. Four types of prayer were identified:

❶ Petitionary prayer: asking for material things you may need.

❷ Ritual prayer: reading the book of prayers.

❸ Meditative prayer: "feeling," or being, in His presence.

❹ Colloquial prayer: talking as to a friend and asking God for guidance in making decisions.

Of all these types of prayer, this study revealed that colloquial prayer correlates best with happiness and religious satisfaction; whereas, ritual prayer was associated with a negative effect producing feelings all the more sad, lonely, tense, and fearful. Talking to God as to a friend, telling Him all our joys and sorrows, can bring happiness, healing, and religious satisfaction. So important is the role of prayer in healing that Dr. Larry Dossey said, "I decided that not to employ prayer with my patients was the equivalent of withholding a potent drug or surgical procedure."[13]

Many people have tried to solve their problems through yoga, secular meditation, or some similar internalized program of self-empowerment; however, these methods do not have the same effectiveness. In many cases they are techniques of self-hypnosis.

SPIRITUAL AND MORAL VALUES

Most civilizations have been founded on a set of beliefs and moral values that lead to an orderly society. Throughout the centuries belief in spiritual values has been a strong motivator to treat others well and to develop peaceful human relationships. History demonstrates that faithless and amoral societies become so corrupt that they cannot survive. Belief is fundamental to science as well as to religion. Just as faith in a scientific principle is verified, faith in God is validated when tests show that its application leads to correct conclusions and brings satisfying results. Studies indicate that those with regular spiritual practices who meet with a faith community live longer, live better, and are far less likely to have a stroke or heart attack. Faith can provide strength to overcome stress

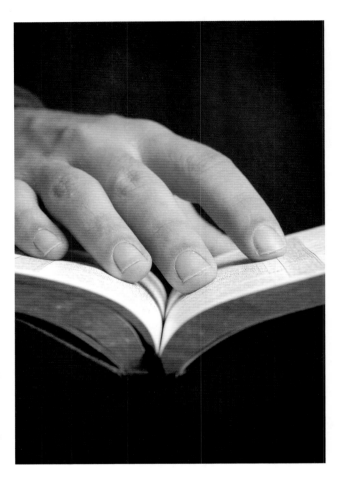

and destructive habits. Belief can give you peace of mind and enable you to reach your full potential through positive choices. Celebrate belief—it is the foundation of life!

PEACE OF MIND

The Bible says, "You will keep him in perfect peace, whose mind is stayed on You, because he trusts in You. (Isa. 26:3, NKJV). When we have a close relationship with God, we experience peace of mind.

This does not mean that those who believe in God and trust Him implicitly will be free from problems. "Trouble and turmoil may surround us, yet we enjoy a calmness and peace of mind of which the world knows nothing. This inward peace is reflected in a . . . vigorous, glowing experience that stimulates all with whom we come in contact. The peace of the Christian depends not upon peaceful conditions in the world about him but upon the indwelling of the Spirit of God."[14]

As nineteenth-century evangelist Dwight L. Moody is quoted by many as saying:

"Trust in yourself, and you are doomed to disappointment.

"Trust in your friends, and they will die and leave you.

"Trust in money, and you may have it taken from you.

"Trust in reputation, and some slanderous tongue may blast it.

"But trust in God, and you will never be confounded in time or eternity."

Trusting in a loving, powerful God provides us with the ability to enjoy a healthful lifestyle. Belief and faith in God enables Him to fill our lives with abundant peace and joy.

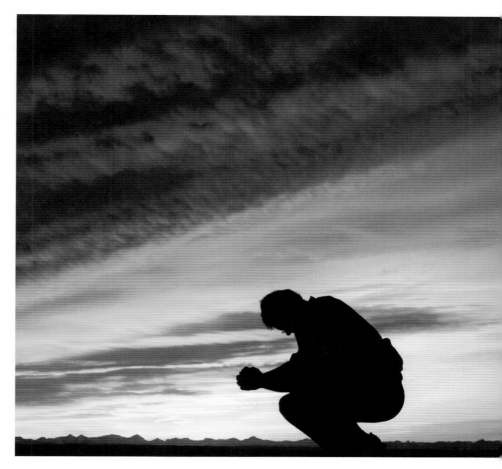

B Celebrating Belief: Life-Application Questions

Take the time to consider these questions and apply what you are learning to your life.

1 How gullible am I? What methods do I use when choosing what to believe? Which influences can I trust: the Internet, advertisements, research backed by vested interests, friends, past experience?

2 What benefits from having faith in God have I noticed? How well have I coped with stressful situations? Do I feel peaceful most of the time? Do I have a strong purpose in life? Is the community in which I live and work aware of this, and are they benefitting, as well? Are adolescents in my community better protected from disruptive and risky behaviors because of my association with them and the faith I exhibit?

3 Which of the four types of prayer do I practice most often? In what ways can I change my prayer habits in order to become more joyful and inwardly peaceful even amid tumultuous events?

GROUP DISCUSSION

4 What are the effects of stress that people experience? How many visits to physicians could be related to not having an ongoing, meaningful relationship of trust with our Savior? How important is it to spend time growing our faith through the study of God's Word and in association with those who have similar beliefs?

5 A classmate of Bruce from academy days stopped attending church. He had a few bad experiences and doubts God's interest in his life situation. In what other ways could Bruce's friend have dealt with that situation? How can Bruce encourage his friend? Would it be helpful to start a fellowship group or small-group Bible study?

Do I need to spend more time growing my faith through the study of God's Word and in association with those who have the same beliefs I do?

Celebrating Rest

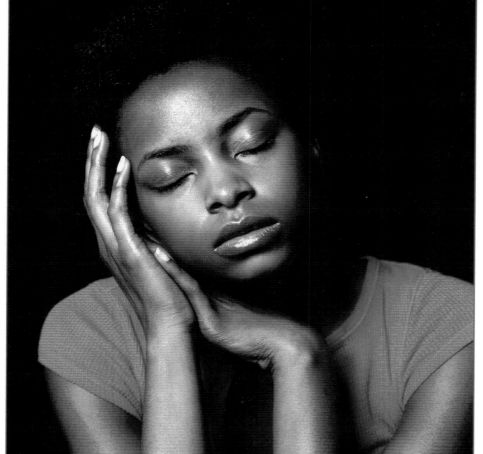

In the United States fatigue is one of the 10 most common reasons people visit a physician.

In 1996, 7-year-old Jessica DuBroff was attempting to be the youngest student pilot to fly across the United States. Accompanying her were her father and her flying instructor. The first couple of days went uneventfully, but as often happens, the media were closely following this attempt and hounded the instructor pilot for midnight and early morning interviews.

While talking with his wife on the phone from Wyoming, the instructor told her how frustrated he was with all the media interruptions, how fatigued he had become as a result of the lost sleep, and how much he was looking forward to being finished with the "media zoo."

The next morning, while preparing for the flight, this instructor with an impeccable record for safety uncharacteristically failed to get a weather briefing before departure. As a result, he flew directly into a storm and the plane crashed shortly after takeoff. No one survived.

Interviews with ground staff later revealed that this very experienced pilot had started the engine without removing the wheel chocks—something

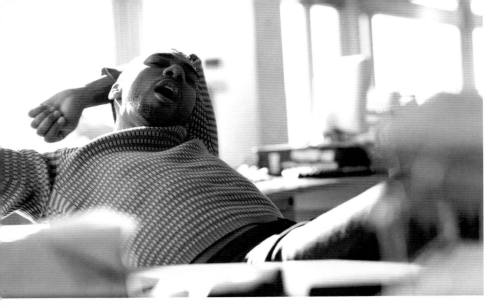
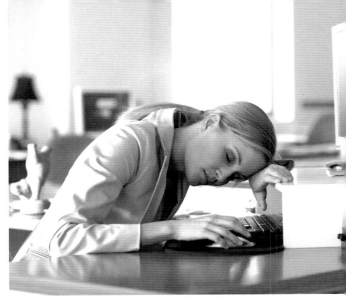
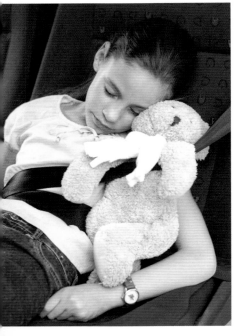
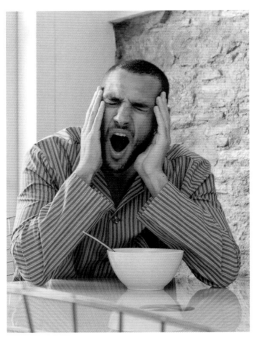
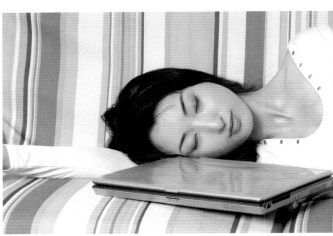
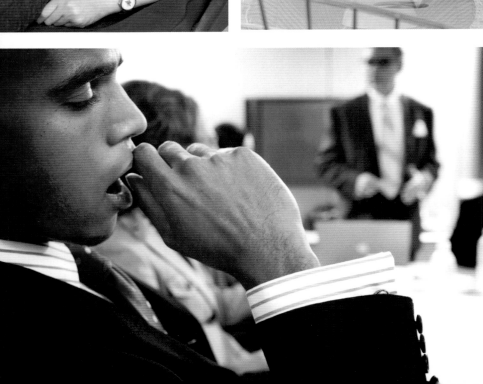
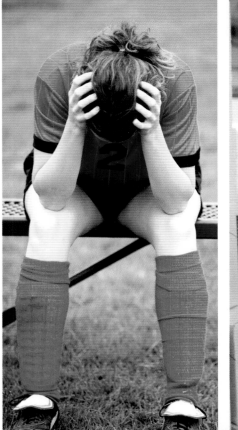
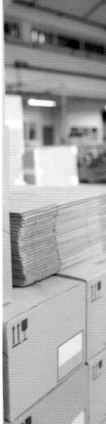

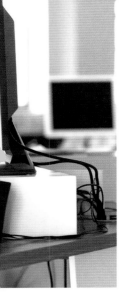

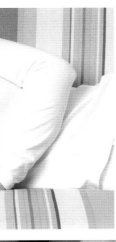

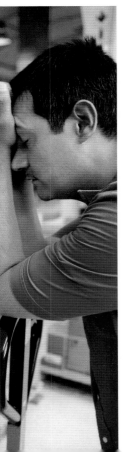

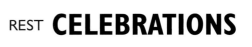

every pilot does before cranking the engine. This forgetfulness evidenced his extreme state of fatigue.*

Sleep science tells us that as in the case of this experienced instructor, tired minds are much more likely to make serious mistakes. In most societies of the world today, a significant percentage of the population is sleep deprived. In the United States fatigue is one of the 10 most common reasons people visit a physician.

The need to rest and relax appears to be the greatest when there seems to be no time for it. Without rest and relaxation all humans suffer cognitive impairments. Tired people become inefficient, slower, less safe, and make more mistakes. To remain "at the top of our game" we need adequate sleep every night. There have been many attempts to increase productivity by extending the workweek and daily working hours. They have all failed because we each have a physiological need for rest each day, as well as a day off each week and a restful annual vacation. For peak cognitive performance and abundant energy, we must celebrate the refreshing gift of sleep.

When our brains are tired enough we will go to sleep involuntarily. These short periods of rest are called micro-sleeps and generally last from a fraction of a second to no more than a second or two. If we are idly sitting in a chair, this usually causes no problem. Should we be operating a complex piece of machinery or carefully seeking to solve a multi-faceted problem, however, these momentary lapses could result in catastrophic outcomes.

SLEEP DEPRIVATION

Many factors of our increasingly chaotic, 24/7 world of tempting and demanding activities contribute to the growing problem of sleep deprivation. The rising number of choices available to us, such as playing computer games or watching television in the evenings, often can delay the onset of sleep. Life has simply become more complex.

A growing body of evidence shows that sleep deprivation impairs our cognitive performance, which in turn influences the quality of our decisions, our emotional control, and our efficiency, productivity, and safety. We all need sufficient rest to restore the wear and tear of life.

Fascinating research has established that when we are tired the "executive functions" of our minds suffer. We become less effective at recognizing the choices that are available to us and less capable of deciding which of the choices is best. Even if we can clearly see the choices, we may not be able to act on what we know we should do. Our creativity is reduced, along with our efficiency.

The frontal lobes of our brains are where we combine the current information from our senses with previously learned information and life ex-

periences to make our decisions. It's this portion of the brain that is most affected by insufficient sleep and rest. Fatigue lowers our cognitive efficiency, lessens the awareness of our surroundings, reduces the ability to process new information, decreases our long-term memory, and impairs the learning of new information. Because success in almost all of life's endeavors is determined by the quality of the decisions we make, it is vitally important to rest as needed.

Sadly, today there is a ubiquitous intrusion of personal, social, and cultural activities into the time that traditionally has been reserved for sleep. Consequently, attention spans are diminished, judgment is impaired, and our ability to carry out complex mental operations is reduced.

SLEEP DEBT

When we miss out on sleep, we accumulate what is known as "sleep debt." As this accumulates, we become less productive. Research was conducted with four groups of people who all had

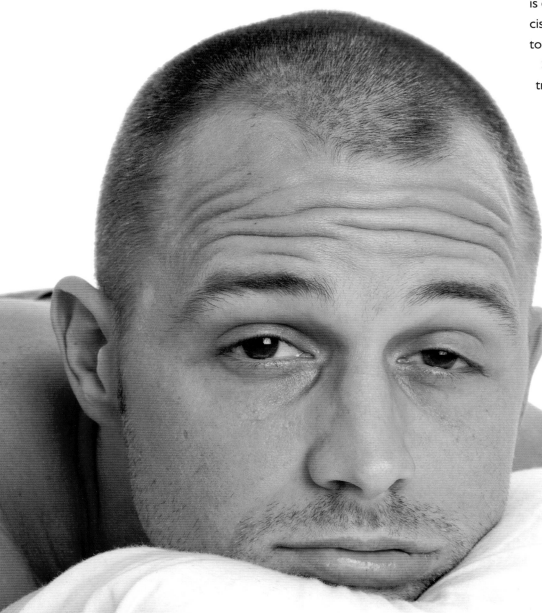

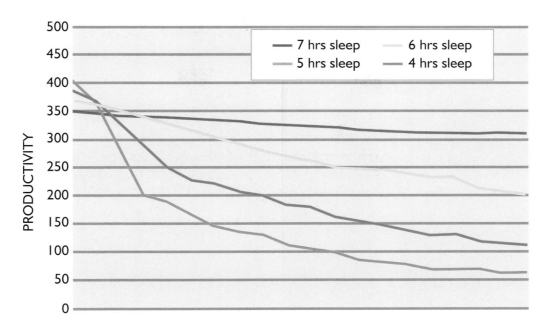

the same demonstrated skill level in performing identical tasks throughout 21 days of activity. The chart above demonstrates how productivity was significantly reduced as nightly sleep was shortened. After the full 21 days of measurements, the productivity of those who got 7 hours of sleep per night dipped about 8 percent. The group that got 6 hours of sleep, however, saw their productivity drop by 55 percent, while those getting 5 and 4 hours of sleep were able to produce only 35 percent and 20 percent respectively of what the 7-hour sleepers produced.

Sleep traditionally has been viewed for its effects on the function of the brain and emotions. Current research, however, is finding that even moderate sleep debt in healthy volunteers can alter their metabolic state in such a way that it mimics the glucose metabolism

of diabetics. After four hours of sleep for six nights, healthy young men experienced a 30-percent decrease in their body's ability to metabolize carbohydrates. They experienced significantly higher levels of the stress hormone cortisol, and a decrease in insulin sensitivity. This and other research is suggesting that there may be a link between the growing epidemic of sleep deprivation and the epidemic of obesity.

It's interesting that sleep deprivation leads to decreased performance similar to that which occurs when a person is under the influence of alcohol. Studies have shown that 16 to 18 hours of wakefulness (one long day) in healthy adults results in impairments comparable to the legal blood-alcohol level of intoxication in the United States and many other countries of greater than 0.08 percent.

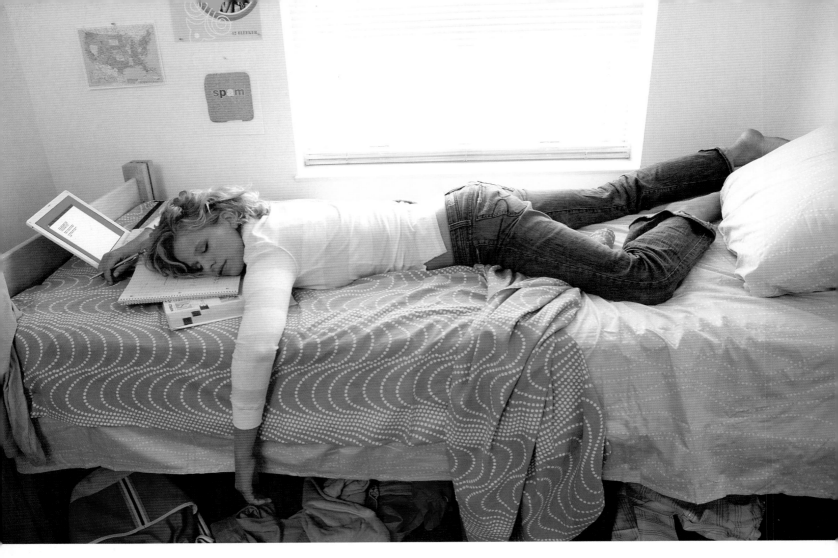

HOW MUCH SLEEP DO WE NEED?

Sleep needs vary between individuals. Nearly all sleep experts agree, however, that seven hours of sleep per night is enough to "get by on," but that most people need about eight hours for optimal cognitive performance. Thomas Edison reportedly believed that sleep was a waste of time, and he set out to invent the electric lightbulb in order to extend daylight hours. He reportedly slept four to five hours per night. Yet, those who worked with him in his laboratory reported that he frequently took naps during the day. Adequate nighttime sleep should remove most daytime sleepiness and provide a sense of calm well-being and alertness.

Students often will study most of the night when cramming for an examination, and they often suffer the consequences of sleep deprivation in poor grades as a result. The way people choose to live and order their lives, along with often hectic work schedules, frequently results in increased inattention at work. Sleep provides the "right stuff." It prepares bodies and minds for peak performance.

STAGES OF SLEEP

Sleep is divided into various stages. These are based on the characteristic

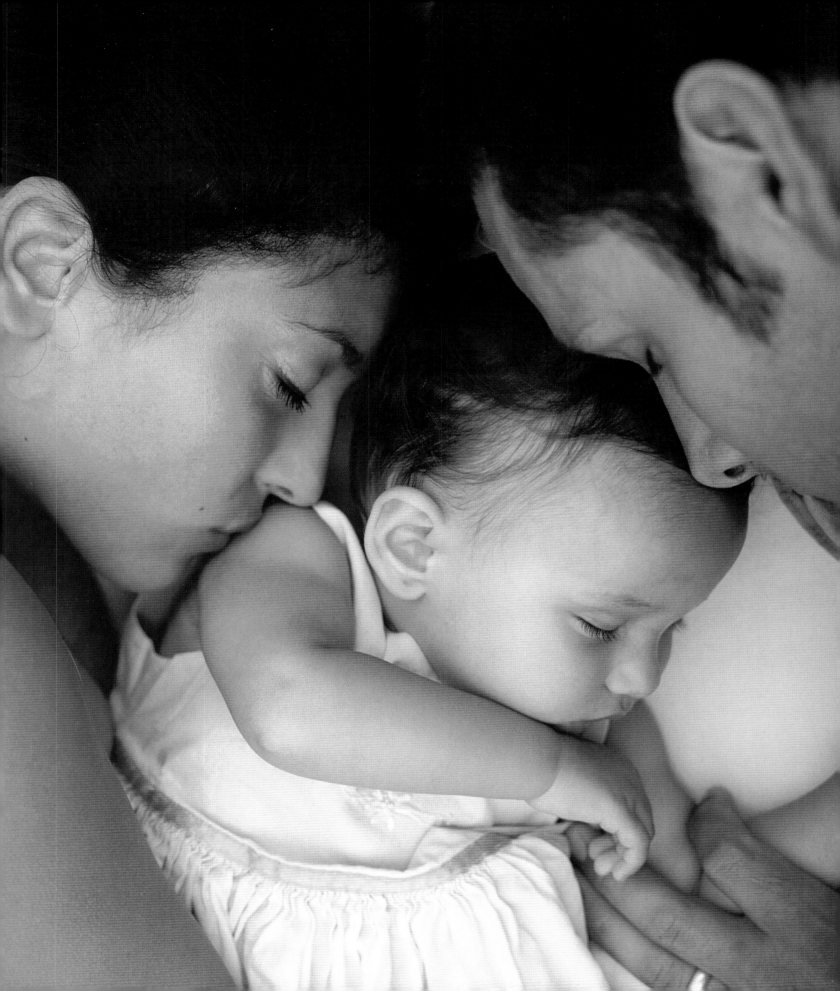

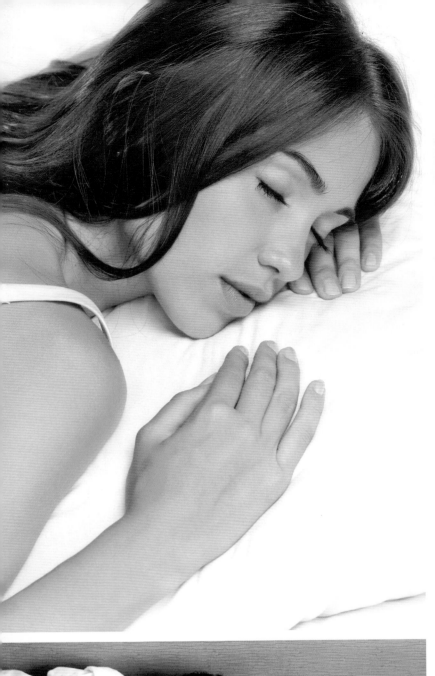

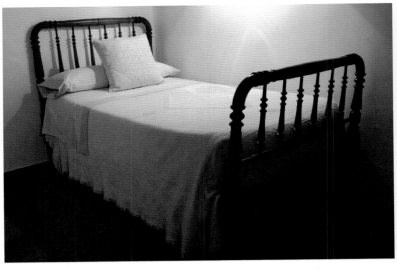

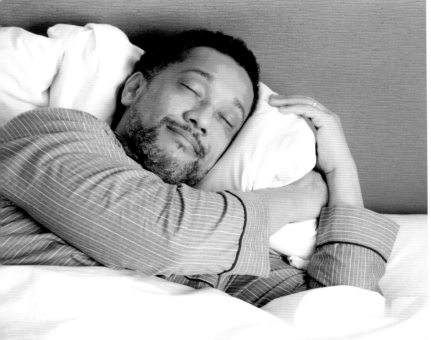

waveforms seen on electro-encephalographic recordings of brain-wave activity. There are two major types of sleep: nonrapid-eye-movement sleep and rapid-eye-movement sleep.

Nonrapid-eye-movement sleep is often characterized by four stages. The first two are deviations from wakefulness and generally last only a few minutes. Stages three and four are known collectively as "slow-wave sleep." It is during this period of "deep sleep" that the restoration and growth of body tissue occur and immunity to infections is strengthened.

Rapid-eye-movement sleep is characterized by a waveform similar to wakefulness. The eyes will move back and forth rapidly under closed lids as though looking from side to side, even though the person is sound asleep. Our dreams occur during this phase of sleep, although we usually recall very little of the dream content. Some individuals may sleep-walk, wet the bed, or grind their teeth during this phase. Rapid-eye-movement sleep is very important for mental and emotional restoration. Many important and fascinating functions take place here, including memory organization and reorganization, as well as the refreshing of memories.

During a good night's sleep, these two types of sleep occur in approximately 90-minute cycles that are repeated from four to six times during the night. Both types of sleep are necessary for complete physical and mental rest. The recuperative value of sleep can be measured by the shape of these cycles and is called the "sleep archi-

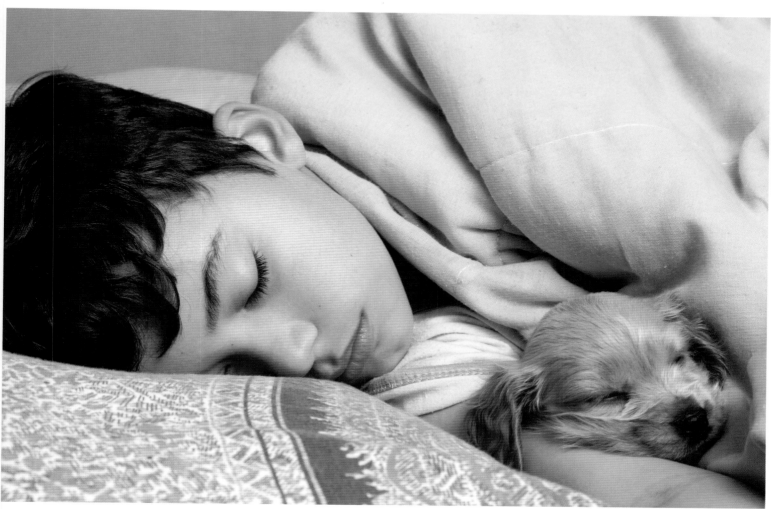

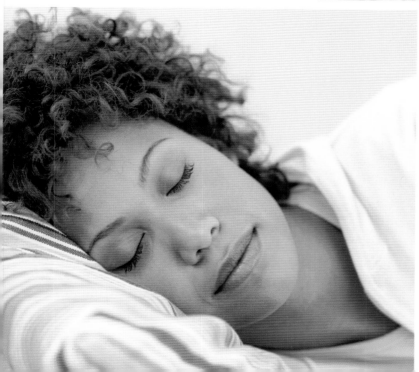

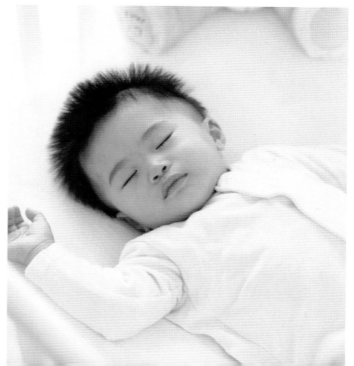

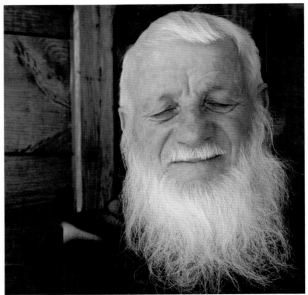

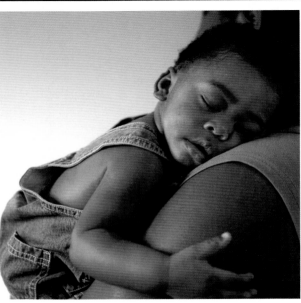

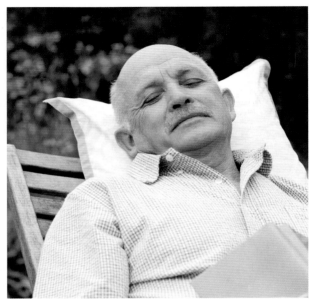

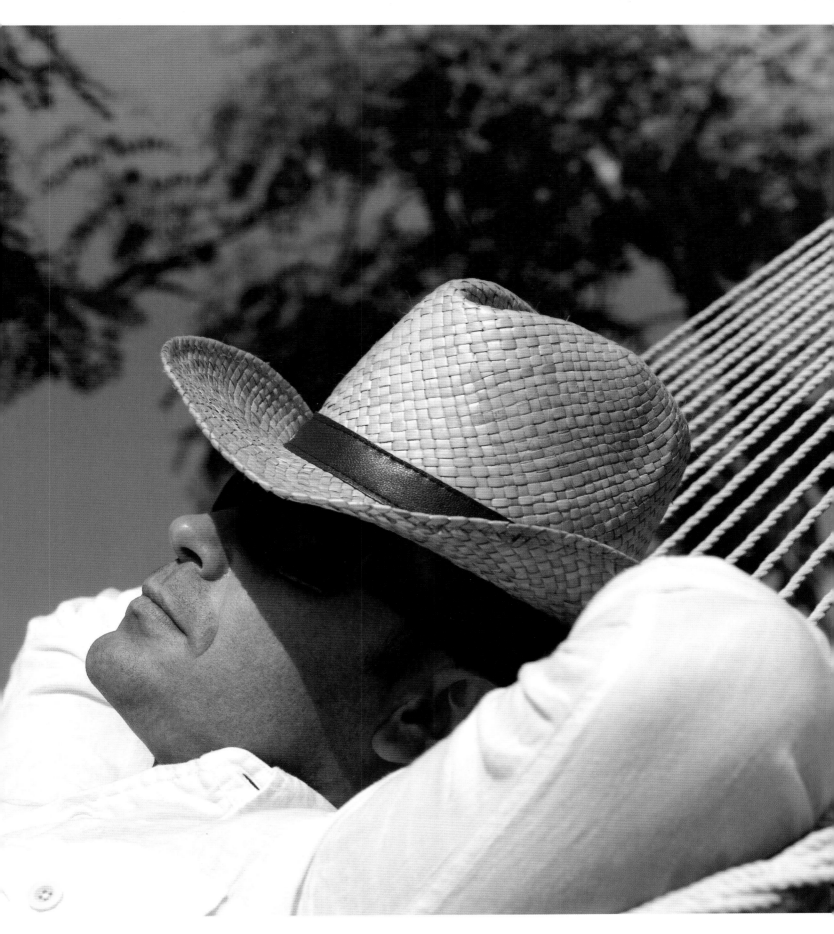

tecture." Good sleep architecture results in recuperative sleep, which enhances learning and improves productivity.

Certain choices—such as irregular times for retiring and awaking, worry and anxiety, certain medications and alcohol, and eating just before going to bed—can impair good architecture.

Sadly, most sleep-deprived people are totally unaware of their own reduced capabilities because they have been sleepy for so long they don't know what it's like to feel wide awake. A rested person will accomplish more in less time and do it better, more effectively, and safely!

STEPS TO GETTING A GOOD NIGHT'S SLEEP

■ Learn to value sleep. We never accomplish what we do not value.

■ Establish a regular bedtime ritual to let your mind and body know that you are preparing to sleep.

■ Exercise appropriately every day, at least four to five hours prior to retiring.

■ Establish regular times for rising and retiring, and stick to them every day—even on weekends.

■ Use a comfortable, firm bed located in a quiet, cool bedroom not cluttered with TVs, computers, and exercise equipment.

■ Eat lightly in the evening, several hours prior to bedtime.

■ Avoid watching exciting or depressing TV programs or movies, engaging in stressful events such as arguments, or making momentous decisions soon before bedtime.

■ Avoid the use of sleeping medications, caffeine, and alcohol, which disrupt normal sleep architecture.

■ See your personal physician if you suspect a sleep disorder or other medical condition.

■ Put your trust in God. Give Him your problems and anxieties.

Remember: Tonight's sleep builds tomorrow's energy! Sleep is as important as diet and exercise, only easier!

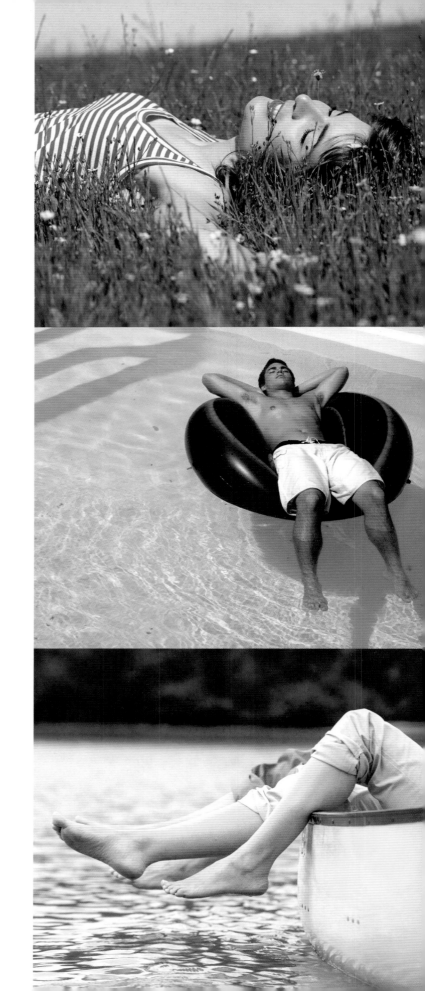

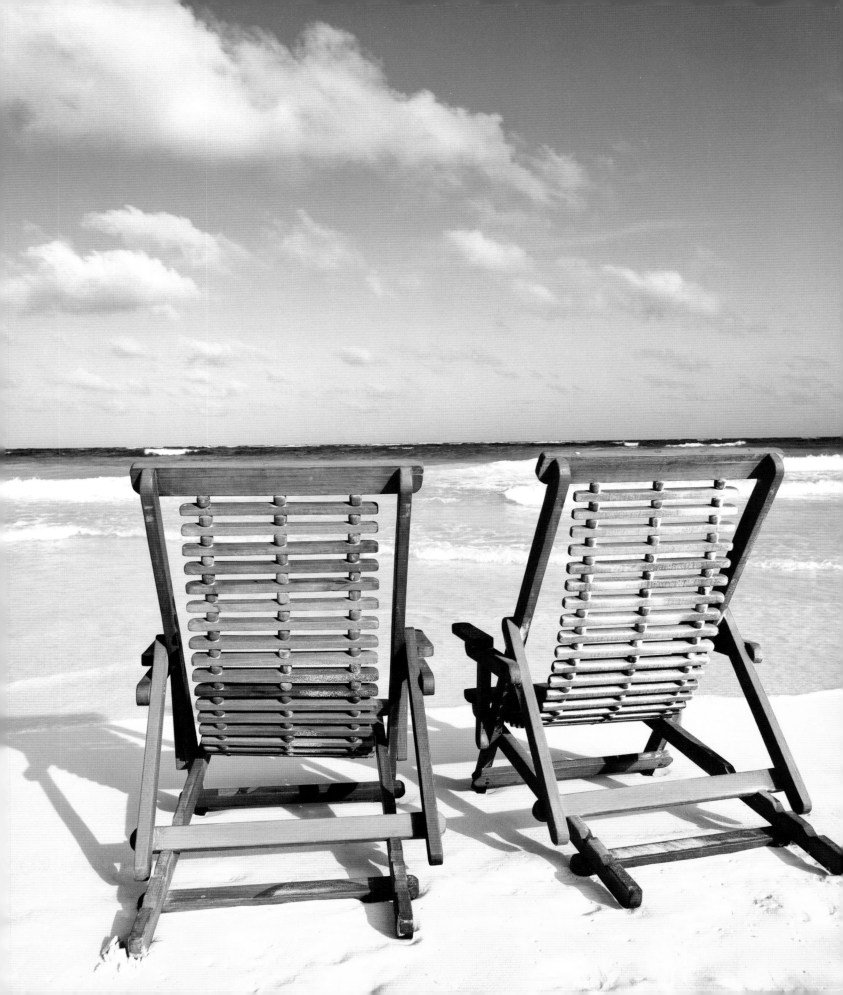

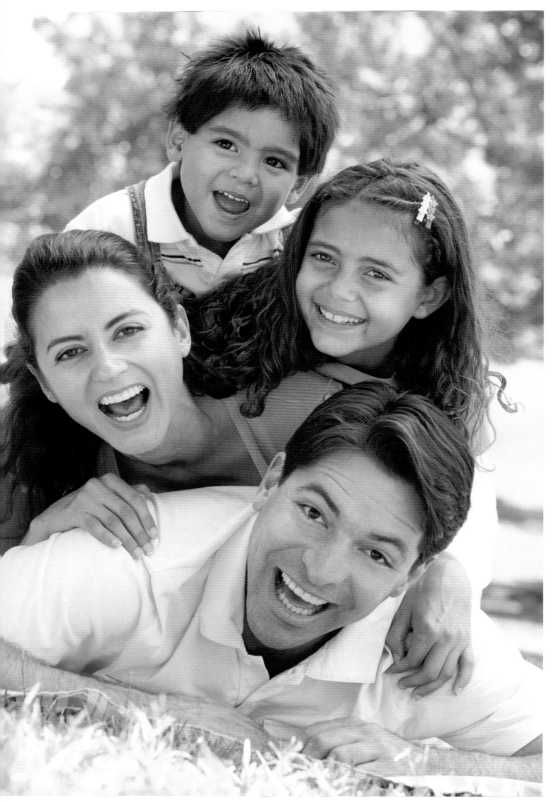

WEEKLY AND ANNUAL REST

Sleep scientists also recognize that to truly remain rested and productive we need both a weekly and an annual rest. In Britain during World War I, increased productivity was attempted by continuous, nonstop work schedules. It was later recognized, however, that by reducing the workweek to 48 hours and requiring one day of rest per week, productivity actually increased by 15 percent.

On July 29, 1941, Winston Churchill announced before the House of Commons, "If we are to win this war it will be by staying power. For this reason we must have one holiday per week and one week holiday per year." That was voted into law!

As humans, we all have our limitations. We cannot work around the clock or without regular times of rest and maintain a healthy, happy, and productive life. We need daily rest as much as we need weekly and annual breaks to provide the mental and emotional recuperation necessary for creativity and positive family relationships. Optimal physical, mental, emotional, and spiritual health require adequate rest.

REST INSTITUTED BY GOD

The Bible records that in the very beginning God instituted a weekly rest to provide a much-needed break from the tedium of work. Our Creator knew that in order to function optimally we need balanced daily rest in addition to weekly rest as found in Exodus 20:8-10: "Remember the Sabbath day, to keep it holy. Six days you shall labor and do all your work, but the seventh day is the Sabbath of the Lord your God. In it you shall do no work: you, nor your son, nor your daughter, nor your male servant, nor your female servant, nor your cattle, nor your stranger who is within your gates."

The Lord wants us to fellowship with Him, especially on the Sabbath day, because He created us as His children. Part of the blessing of the Sabbath rest comes as we support and relate with others during these special hours. Christ said in Mark 2:27, "The Sabbath was made for man, and not man for the Sabbath" (NKJV).

Daily sleep and a weekly rest empower us to be receptive to the blessings of God physically, mentally, emotionally, socially, and spiritually, thus continually restoring us to optimal health.

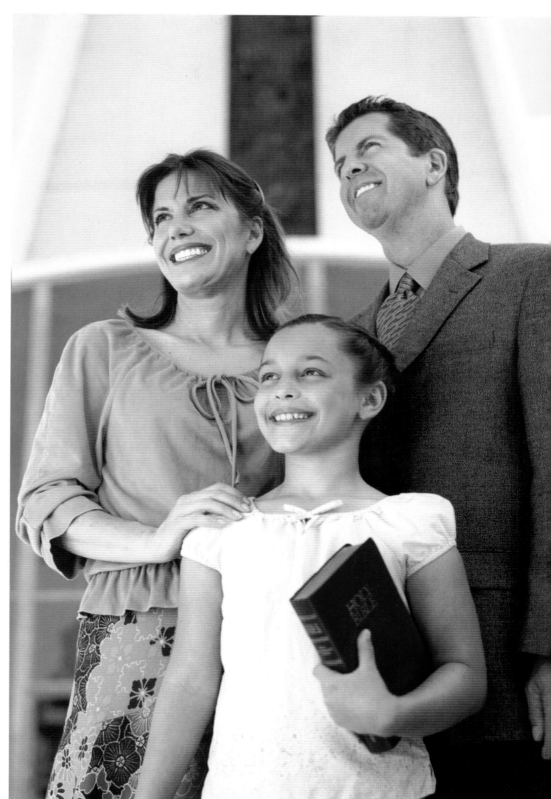

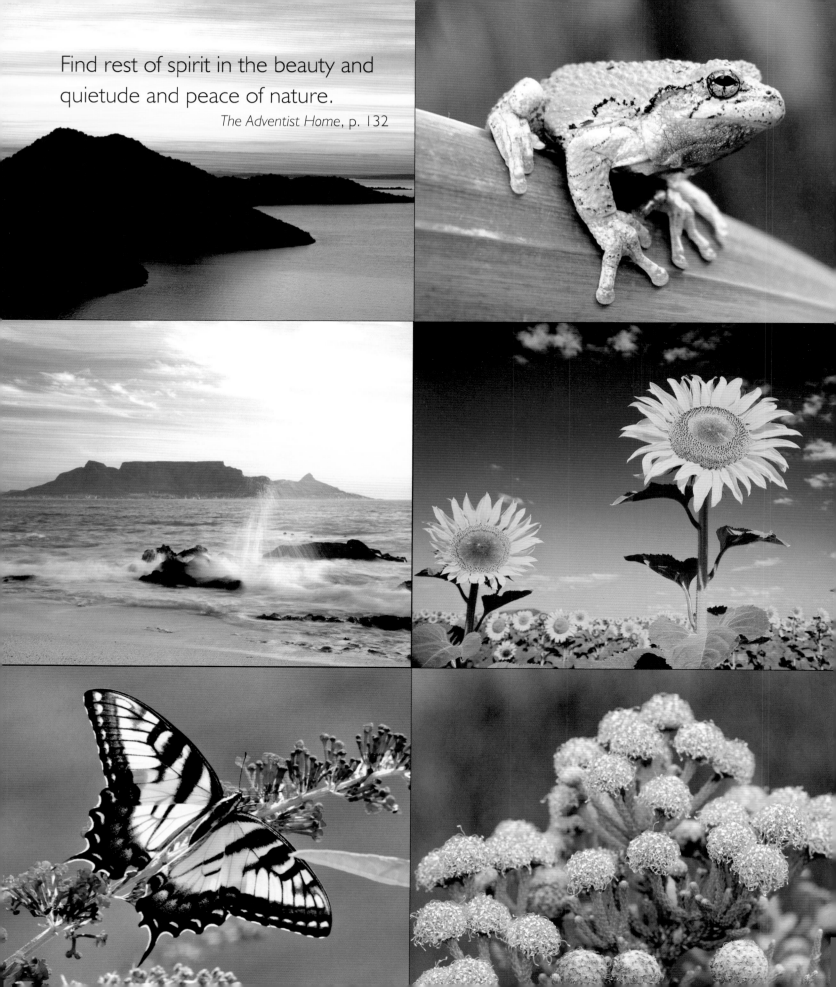

Find rest of spirit in the beauty and quietude and peace of nature.

The Adventist Home, p. 132

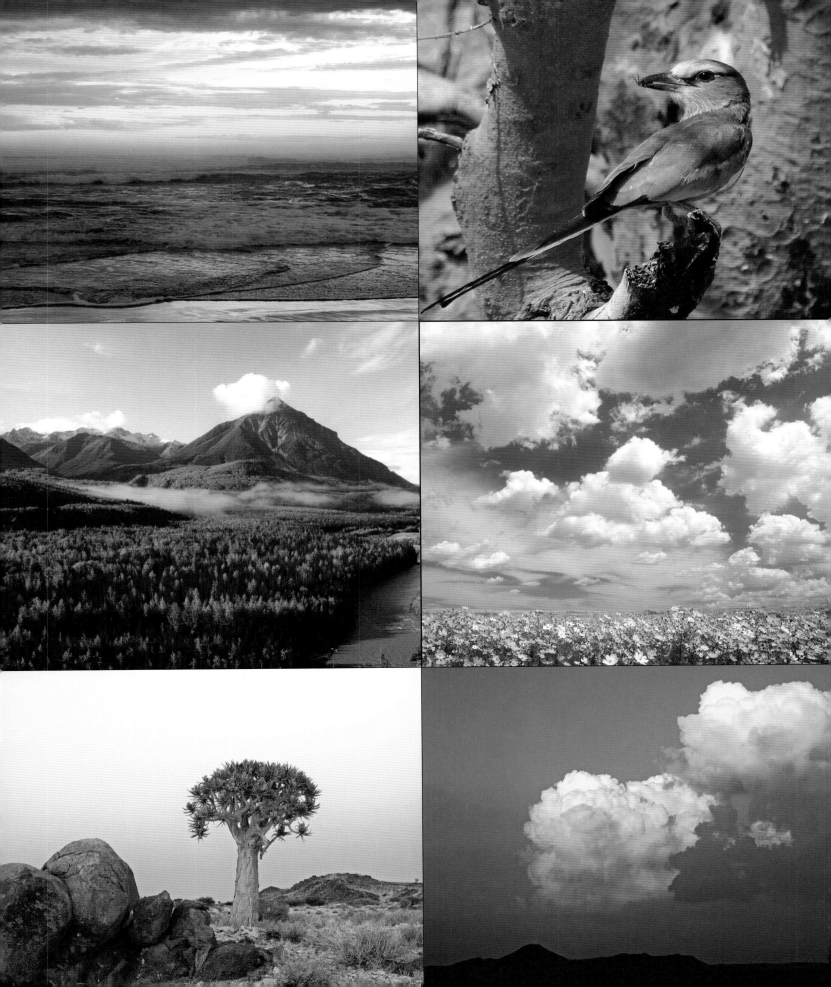

Celebrating Rest: Life-Application Questions

Take the time to consider these questions and apply what you are learning to your life.

1 How many times in the last three days have I fallen asleep involuntarily? How many hours of nightly sleep have I had during that same time? Do I need to reassess my sleeping habits? Am I staying up too late at night? What delays my preparation for bed? Do I need to exercise more, or perhaps earlier in the day? Have I had too big a meal in the evening, or eaten too late? Am I worrying about something that is keeping me awake? Am I choosing to watch too much TV or play too many games? Do I need to see my physician about a sleep disorder, such as sleep apnea?

2 How many of the following symptoms have I observed in myself lately: lower productivity; short attention span; bad judgment calls; inability to solve complex problems, think clearly, or remember quickly?

3 How do I demonstrate that I value my sleep? What choices do I have to make in order to get adequate and restful sleep? Should I choose to get up at the same time on weekends as I do during the week so that I establish good-habit patterns? What arrangements in my bedroom do I have to change to foster better sleep? How can I make a decided choice to put my trust in God and leave my burdens with Him?

GROUP DISCUSSION

4 A husband and wife worked late and then went out to dinner with friends. The meal was delicious, but the couple ate too much. Neither slept well when they eventually got to bed. The next evening they arrived home late again and then watched a late-night TV show. The next morning the couple had a heated argument about who should fetch the dry cleaning. Why would they argue about such an inconsequential thing? Were they thinking clearly? How can such irritable feelings be prevented?

5 In what ways do we show that we value the rest that the Sabbath offers? Should we use Sabbath hours to catch up on sleep debt from a week of bad choices? Or should we enjoy the same type of rest that God took after Creation—a rest from work in order to spend time in growing our relationships with God, family, and community?

6 Do we use the full vacation time allotted to us? How can we best use this time in a balanced way to adequately rejuvenate physically, mentally, emotionally, and spiritually? How can we plan more purposefully to gain the benefits we need to offset the stresses and deficiencies we experience during the rest of the year?

Should I choose to get up at the same time on weekends as I do during the week so that I establish good-habit patterns?

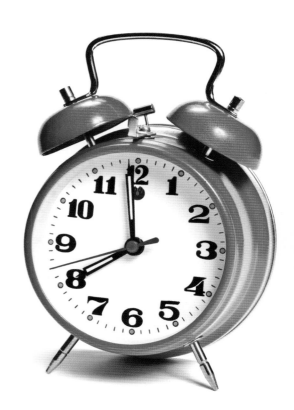

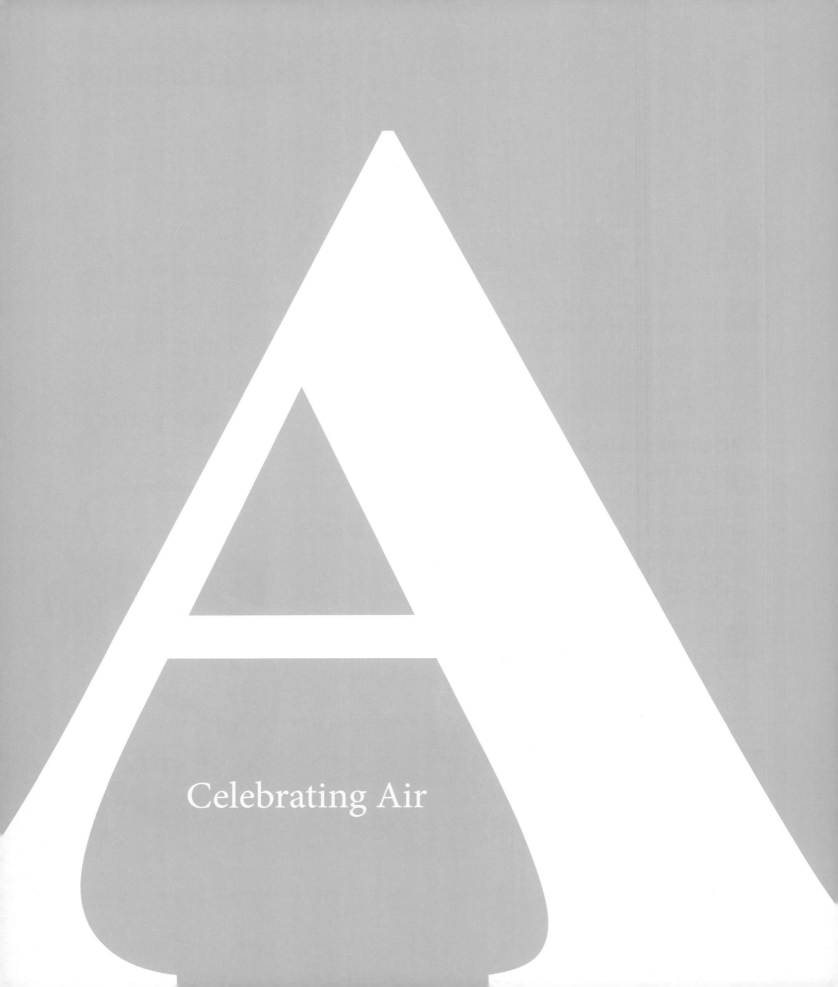

Celebrating Air

The rush of air that whipped passed their faces was invigorating! It didn't matter that the temperature was near freezing. Orville was guiding the first controlled flight, and his brother, Wilbur, was running alongside the wing of the flying machine. It was December 17, 1903, and the Wright brothers made a total of four short but historic flights.

Experiencing the success of such a momentous achievement made the practice runs, the hard work, and the criticism of the skeptics pale into insignificance. Apart from the sheer dogged determination of the Wright brothers and the foundational experience of other aviation pioneers such as Otto Lilienthal, without the air and its physical properties providing the "lift," flight never would have taken place. Lift is a complex physical phenomenon that enables birds and airplanes to fly. Other properties of air allow living creatures to breathe and exist.

Those early flight experiences kindle feelings in us of excitement and

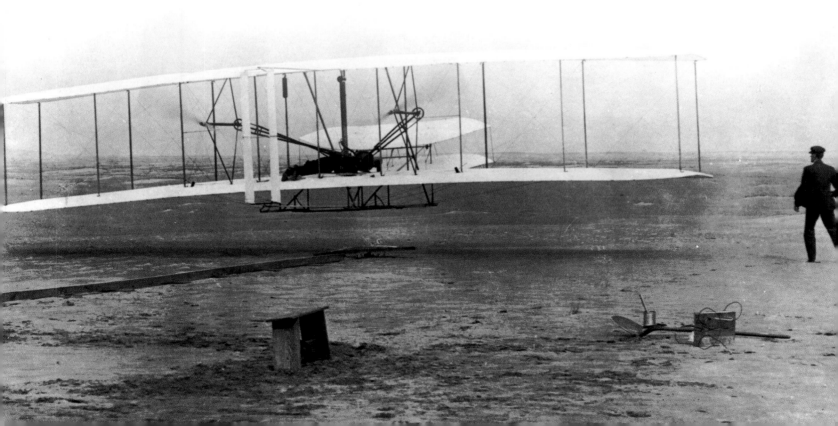

exhilaration. In contrast, some other events elicit discouragement and despair. Shortly after midnight on December 3, 1984, in the city of Bhopal, India, for example, a poisonous gas cloud escaped from a pesticide factory. The toxic gas covered an area of 30 square miles, immediately killing thousands of people and causing illness for many more. Experts believe that as time went on, many more people eventually perished as a result of this environmental disaster and the severe air pollution that ensued. Clean air is essential and literally constitutes the physical breath of life.

HOW DOES IT WORK?

Atmospheric air comprises a mixture of gases: 20.98 percent oxygen (O_2), 0.04 percent carbon dioxide (CO_2), 78.06 percent nitrogen (N_2), and 0.92 percent inert (inactive) constituents such as argon and helium. Oxygen is the vital component of air that sustains life. Breathing is the process that moves the air in and out of the lungs and continues the cycle of taking in oxygen and releasing carbon dioxide. This process takes in and exchanges approximately 20,000 liters (5,283 gallons) of air daily. The body carries approximately 1.89 liters (2 quarts) of oxygen in the lungs, blood, and other tissues at any given time. Once oxygen enters the lungs, it goes into the bloodstream by a process called diffusion. The heart and circulatory system then pump the blood to every tissue of the body, delivering life-giving oxygen to the tissues and cells. Oxygen promotes efficient cell function by facilitating the metabolism of nutrients and the transfer of energy within the cells.

The exchange of gases in the lungs occurs across a thin wall approximately two cells thick. These cells line the tiny air sacs of the lungs (alveoli) and also the small blood vessels (capillaries), which carry the oxygen-rich blood to the rest of the body. The waste carbon dioxide is released into the air sacs and expelled from the lungs. The oxygen is carried by millions of red blood cells, which nourish all the body tissues and cells. The exchange of oxygen and carbon dioxide is accomplished within milliseconds, and it takes about only one minute for the newly acquired oxygen to circulate through the body! The lungs are wonderfully designed in order to reach this efficiency and contain more than 600 million of these alveoli (air sacs).

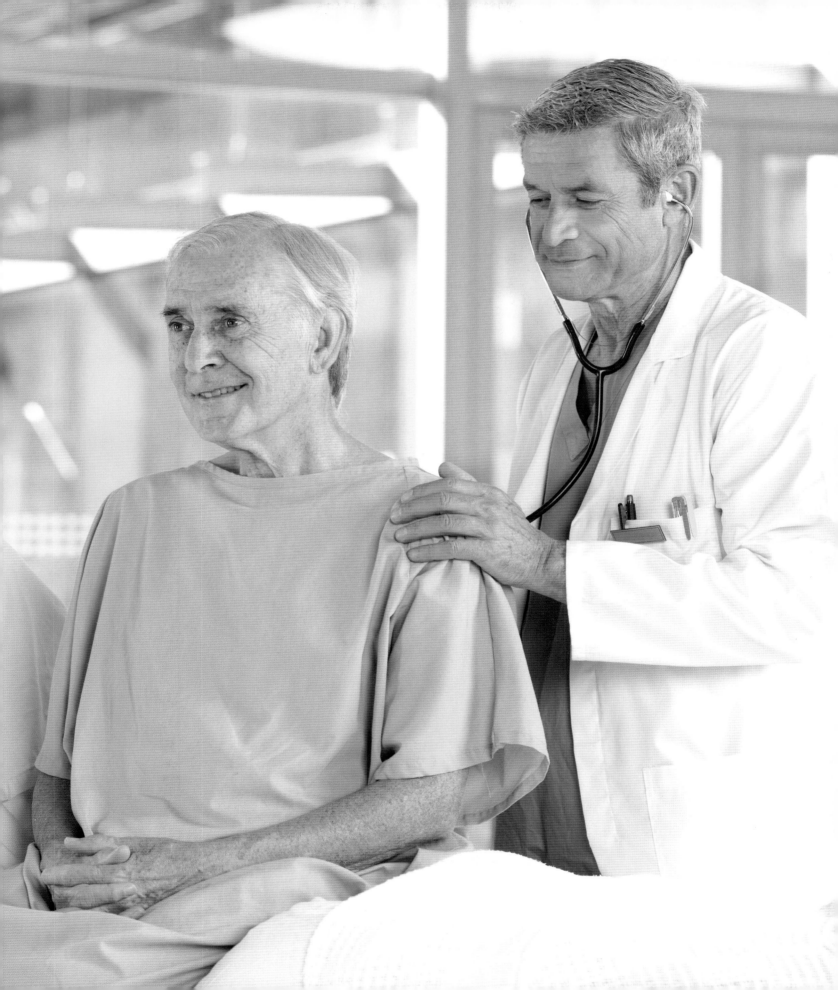

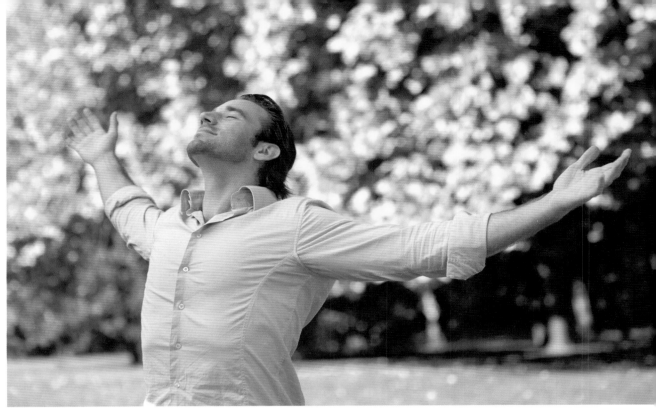

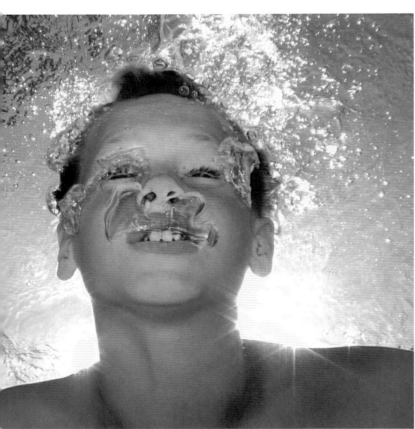

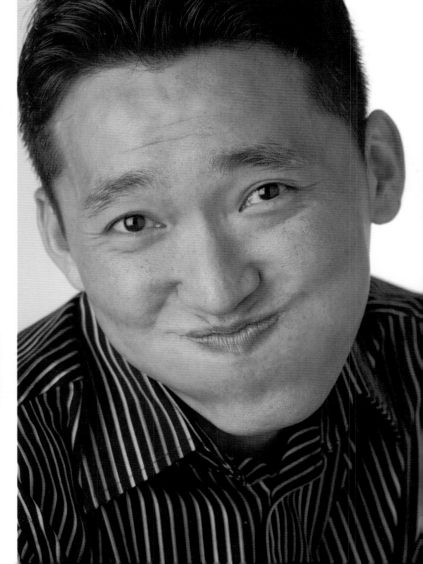

The body ensures normal oxygen levels (saturation) by driving the respiration (breathing rate) from a part of the brain called the medulla oblongata in the brain stem. These specialized brain centers automatically regulate the rate and depth of breathing according to the needs of the body while carbon dioxide levels play a very important role in stimulating breathing. It is for this reason that it's not possible for a healthy person to voluntarily stop breathing for prolonged, indefinite time periods. If one does not inhale fresh air, the level of carbon dioxide builds up in the blood, resulting in the feeling of tremendous "air hunger" forcing one to breathe. This miraculous, irrepressible reflex is lifesaving; if breathing stops, the body's oxygen levels drop dangerously low within minutes, leading to permanent brain damage, followed by death. Brain cells begin to die within four minutes of oxygen deprivation. This fact emphasizes the accuracy of the American Lung Association's motto, "It's a matter of life and breath." We need oxygen for life, and pure fresh air for health.

HOW DOES EXERCISE CHANGE THINGS?

During exercise, the increased cellular activity of the muscles produces more carbon dioxide. The carbon dioxide acts on specialized receptors and the respiration center in the brain, causing a higher rate of respiration, which is also deeper. During rest, the breathing rate is lower because the carbon dioxide production is lower. Control mechanisms, however, ensure adequate breathing to provide appropriate amounts of oxygen to all body cells. In addition to removing carbon dioxide from the body, breathing results in a loss of water from the body in the form of water vapor. This is one of the forms of "invisible" water loss, so named because it is not seen or obvious. Prolonged, rapid, deep breathing can aggravate dehydration; this may occur in prolonged exercise, heat exhaustion, and disease states.

We need oxygen for life, and pure fresh air for health.

131

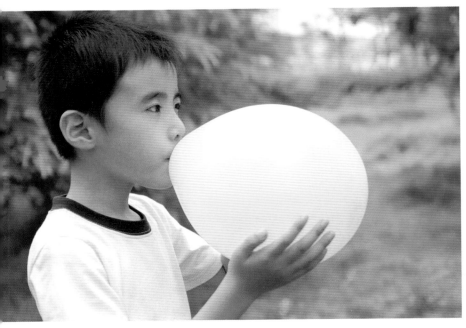

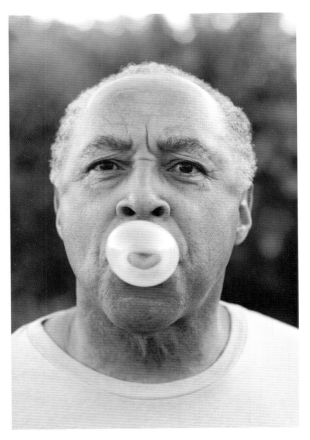

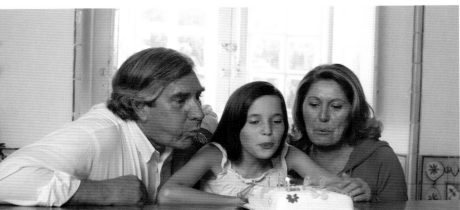

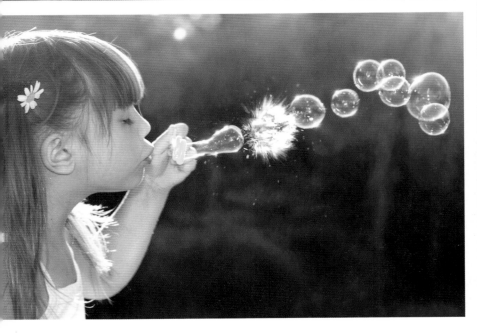

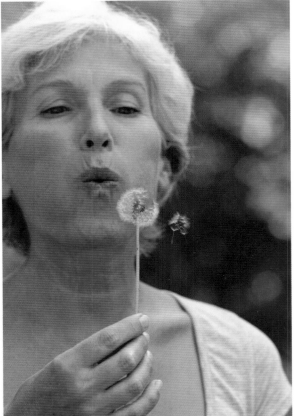

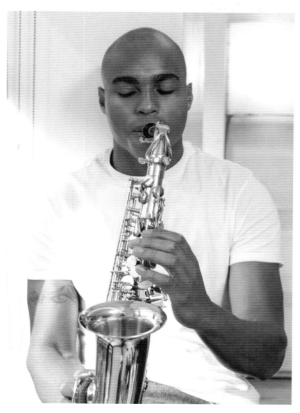
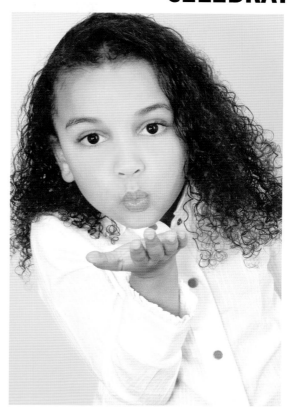
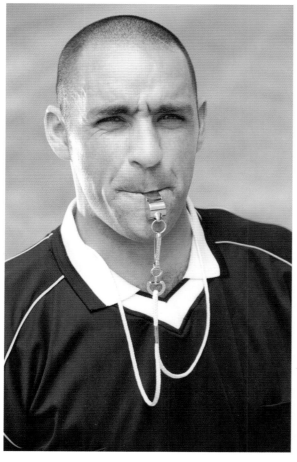
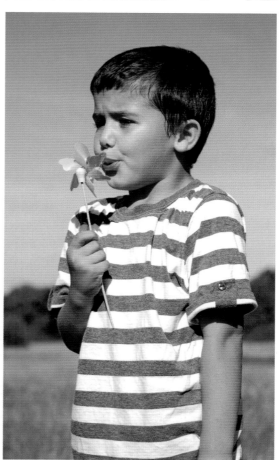

DON'T SKIMP ON QUALITY

High-quality fresh air is pure and clean. The life-giving oxygen molecules should be unpolluted. Deep breathing of fresh air imparts an improved sense of well-being. It increases the rate and quality of growth in plants and animals. It improves the function of the lung's protective cilia. These are the microscopic, fine, hair-like structures that help to keep dust and fine particles as well as irritants from entering the lungs. Good oxygenation lowers the body temperature and resting heart rate, and decreases the survival of certain bacteria and viruses found in the air.

Fresh air is often destroyed and polluted. This can occur through inadequate ventilation of dwellings, especially where open cooking fires and stoves are used. In cities the air in buildings is often recirculated through air-conditioning systems, increasing the pollution from city smog, tobacco smoke, and industrial and other pollutants. On the other hand, good quality air usually can be found in abundance in natural outdoor environments, especially around trees (sometimes called the "lungs of the earth"); green plants; mountains and forests; lakes, oceans, rivers, and waterfalls; and after rainfall. It's estimated that the algae in the ocean provide almost 90 percent of the oxygen in our atmosphere, with the rest coming from land plants.

Fresh air, when unpolluted, is invigorating! Notice how exhilarated you feel near a waterfall or at the ocean. This may be one of the reasons for the popularity of holiday resorts and vacation areas in the mountain areas and at the seaside.

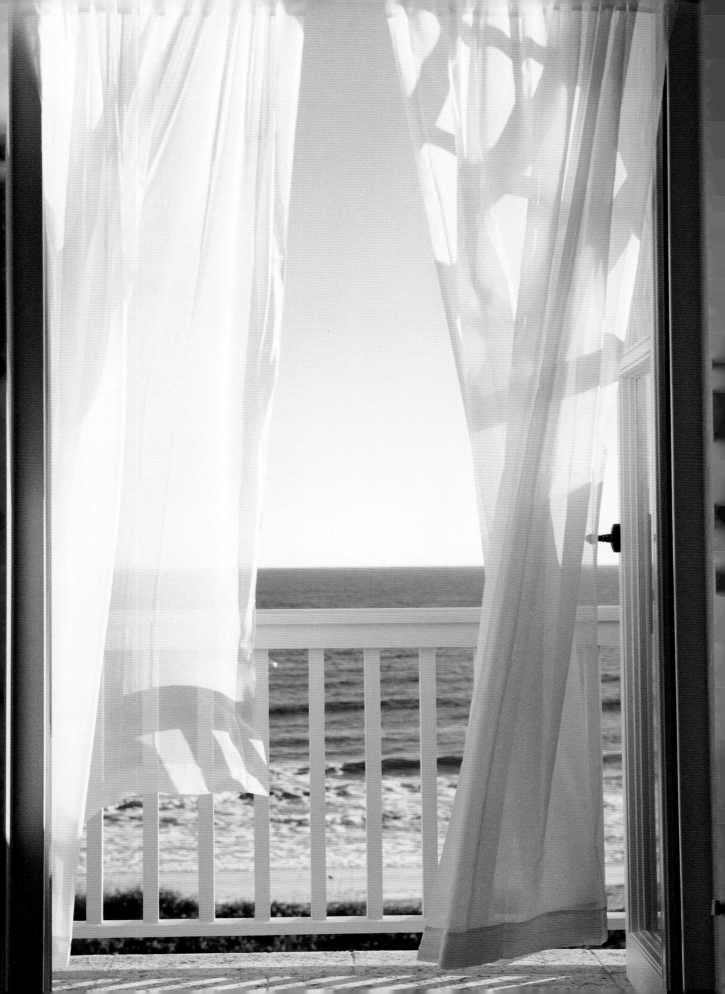

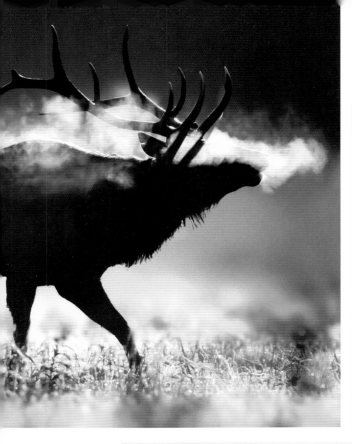

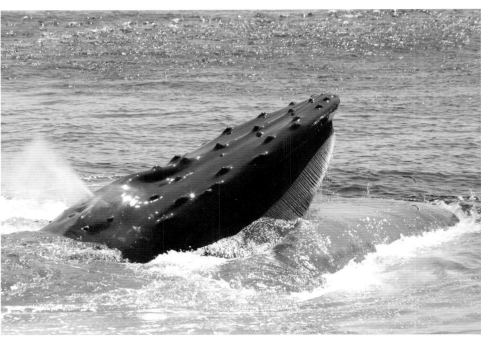

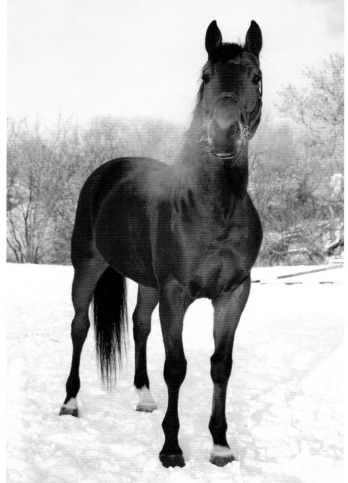

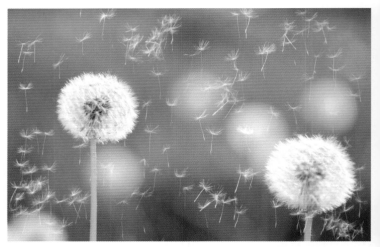

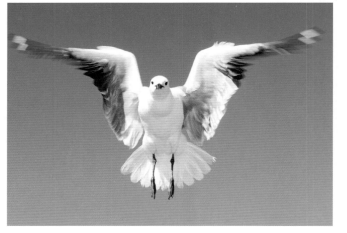

In his hand is the life of every creature and the breath of all mankind. Job 12:10, NIV

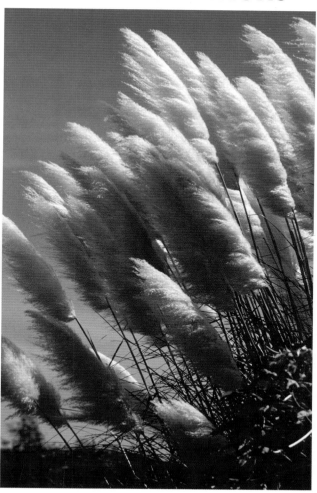

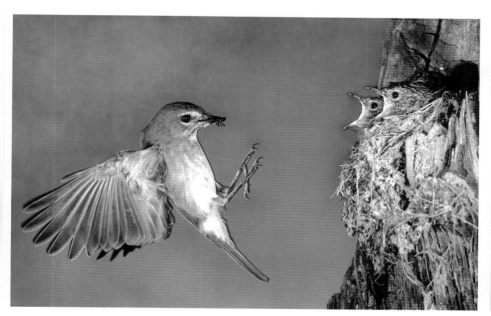

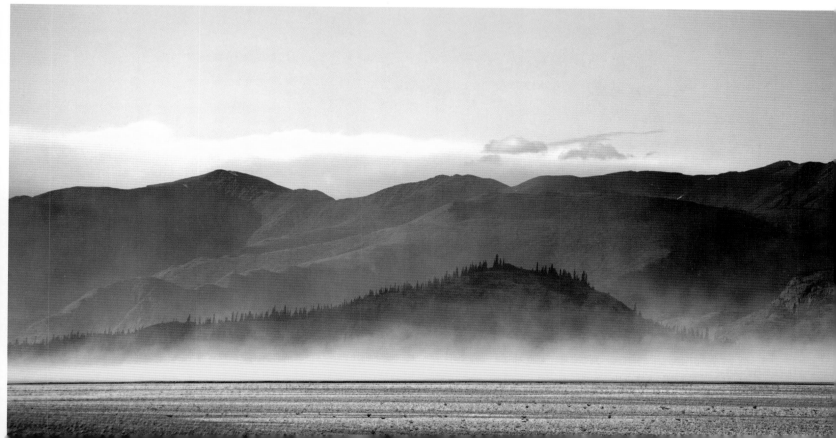

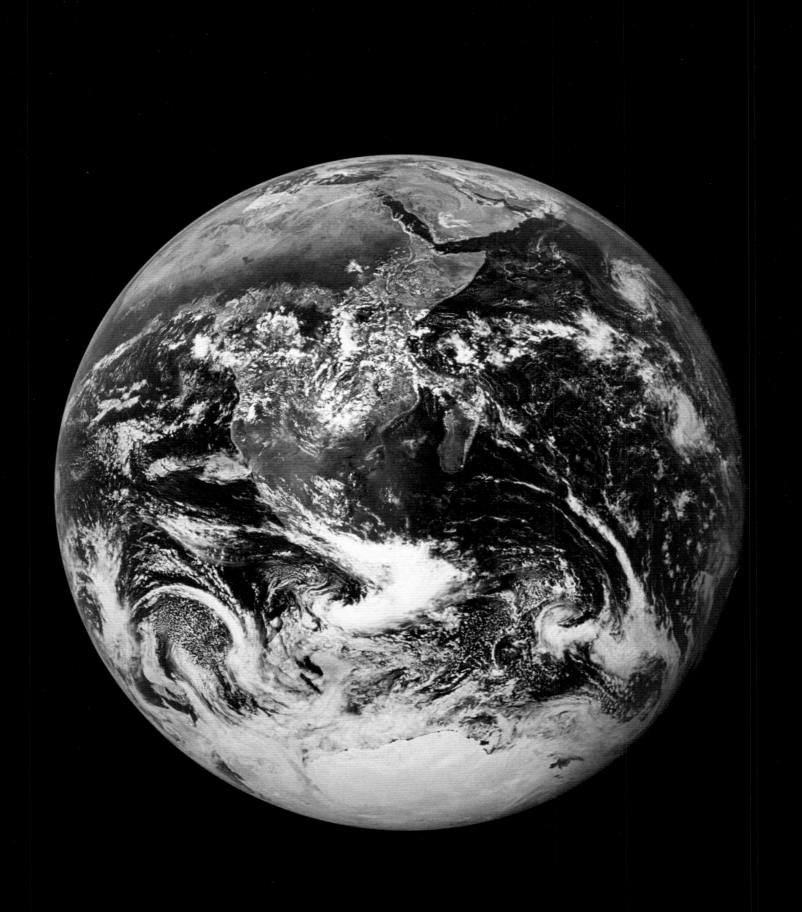

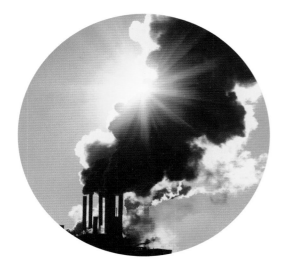

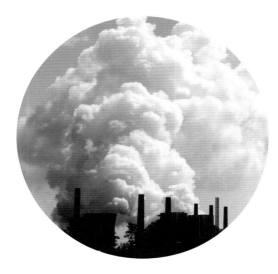

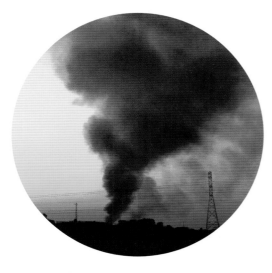

PROTECTING OUR INTERESTS

The air also has many protective qualities. On a global level the air and its suspended water vapor protect the earth and its inhabitants from solar radiation and the cold vacuum of outer space. The air recycles water and many chemicals to moderate the climate. Within this atmospheric envelope, life is found over a very wide range of altitudes and temperatures. Some life-forms require large amounts of oxygen; others only a scant amount. For humans to have optimal health, fresh, clean air is essential.

AIR POLLUTION

Polluted air is found on freeways, at airports, and in closed, poorly ventilated areas. Polluted, smoke-filled air can be associated with increased anxiety, migraine headaches, nausea, vomiting, eye problems, irritability, and respiratory congestion. The World Health Organization (WHO) estimates that more than 2 million people die every year from breathing in tiny pollutant particles present in indoor and outdoor air pollution. These tiny particles, called PM-10 particles (10 micrometers or less), can penetrate the lungs and may enter the bloodstream causing heart disease, lung cancer, asthma, and acute lower respiratory infections.[1] Some 6 million people, mostly children, die each year from acute respiratory infections, complicated particularly by indoor pollution often originating from unvented or poorly vented cooking facilities. In many cities the PM-10 particle level is 15 times above the recommended safety guidelines. The evidence that air pollution results in increased strokes and vascular disease including heart attacks is growing. Additionally, researcher Jennifer Weuve and colleagues have shown that long-term exposure to air pollution speeds up cognitive decline in older women and may increase the progression to dementia.[2,3,4]

The results of pollution described above are sometimes beyond the control of the individual. This is often the case for the "passive smoker," one who is exposed to secondhand tobacco smoke. Children frequently are victims of secondhand smoke (SHS) in homes where parents and other family members smoke. These children have an increased risk of suffering lower respiratory tract infections and middle ear infections.[5] The severity and number of asthma episodes in asthmatic children are increased by exposure to SHS. There also is evidence linking tobacco smoke pollution to increased Sudden Infant Death Syndrome (SIDS).[6] Adults exposed to SHS have an increased risk of lung cancer estimated at 20 percent in women and 30 percent in men who live with a smoker.[7] Smoke pollution in the workplace increases the risk of nonsmokers developing lung cancer by 16 to 19 percent.

WHAT TO DO?

What can we do to ensure that we get adequate amounts of clean air and vital oxygen? Avoid tobacco smoke, and, as much as possible, stay out of polluted environments. Avoid shallow breathing; take deep breaths and exercise regularly. This helps us to take full advantage of the natural lung capacity and prevents the lower parts of the lung being underventilated. Take intentional breaks during work time to breathe deeply—outdoors, if possible. Good posture and diaphragmatic breathing also are helpful in obtaining optimal respiration, ventilation, and blood flow through the lungs.

Good posture: The late Dr. Mervyn Hardinge, dean emeritus of Loma Linda University School of Public Health, suggested these five steps to help individuals acquire good posture habits:

1 Flatten the plane of the pelvis by contracting the large gluteus muscles.

2 Stand tall, thus decreasing the forward and backward curves of the spine.

3 Keep the head back, chin horizontal, and eyes looking straight ahead.

4 The feet should be slightly apart and directed forward, the upper limbs hanging naturally by the side.

5 Exercise so as to stretch and strengthen muscles.

Constriction of the thoracic cage by poor posture or even states of disease, often results in diminished lung volume and respiratory reserve. Good posture enhances one's respiratory capacities and exercise capabilities.

Diaphragmatic breathing: People who are fit and exercise regularly also strengthen the muscles of respiration, of which the diaphragm is the most important. To practice diaphragmatic breathing do the following:

1 While standing, stretch your arms high above your head.

2 Breathe in slowly, mouth closed. Normally the lower ribs will expand.

3 Expand the chest as far as possible while breathing in. At the height of inspiration, take one more whiff of air.

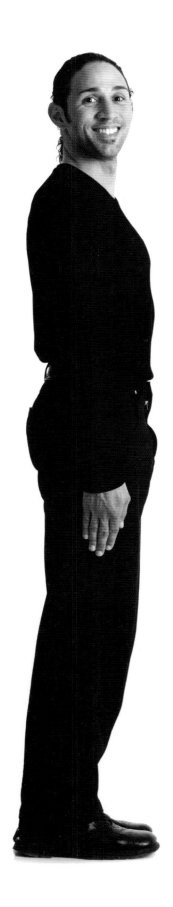

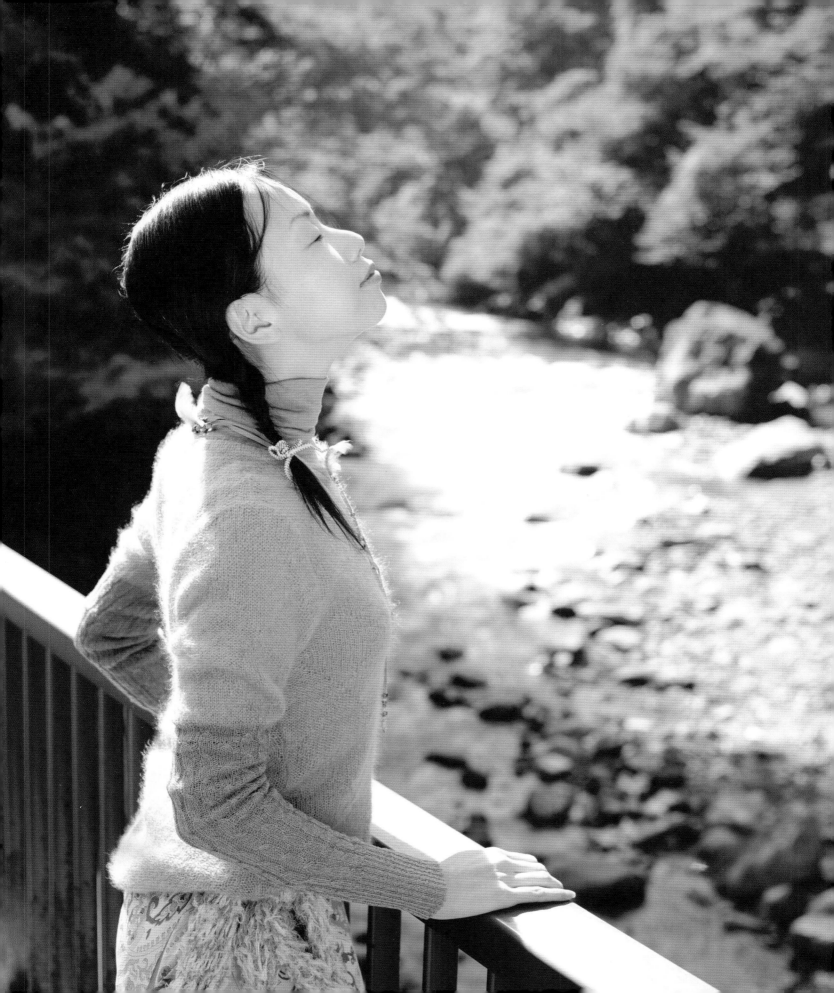

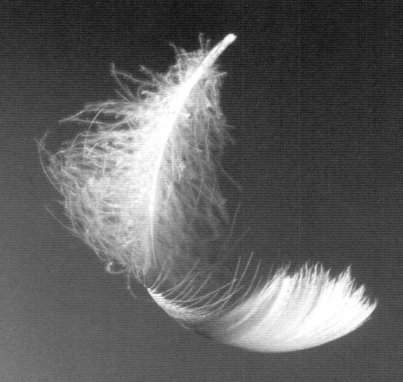

The free, pure air of heaven
is one of the richest blessings
we can enjoy. *Testimonies*, vol. 2, p. 528

4 With mouth open let all the air out while slowly bending over. Cough to get the last bit of air out.

5 Repeat five to ten times every morning.

Diaphragmatic breathing aerates the respiratory tract and reduces the risk of infection. Quiet breathing moves about 500 cubic centimeters of air in and out of the lungs, whereas the total volume that can pass in and out of the lungs in one breath—the vital capacity—is about 4,000 cubic centimeters, eight times greater than during quiet breathing.

The cells most sensitive to lack of oxygen are those of the brain. The brain is the seat of judgment, reason, intellect, and the will—the control center of our entire being. It's essential to ensure optimal oxygenation of the brain by avoiding underventilated areas where carbon dioxide, carbon monoxide, and other pollutants may interfere with normal oxygen availability.

IN THE BEGINNING

The atmosphere surrounding the earth provides our wonderfully designed and created bodies with the literal breath of life. Right in the beginning the Lord God our Creator made this provision to support life: "The Lord God formed man of the dust of the ground, and breathed into his nostrils the breath of life; and man became a living being" (Gen. 2:7, NKJV). We have the privilege and responsibility to ensure that our body receives the purest, freshest air possible. We also need to care for the environment and do all we can, individually and collectively, to prevent and minimize air pollution. We cannot do this alone. We need the sustaining power and grace of the loving creator God.

"In the matchless gift of His Son, God has encircled the whole world with an atmosphere of grace as real as the air which circulates around the globe. All who choose to breathe this life-giving atmosphere will live and grow up to the stature of men and women in Christ Jesus."[8]

As we celebrate a vital and fulfilled life, we need to breathe deeply, exercise well, enjoy the beauty of the great outdoors, and never forget the indwelling presence of God, the Breath of Life.

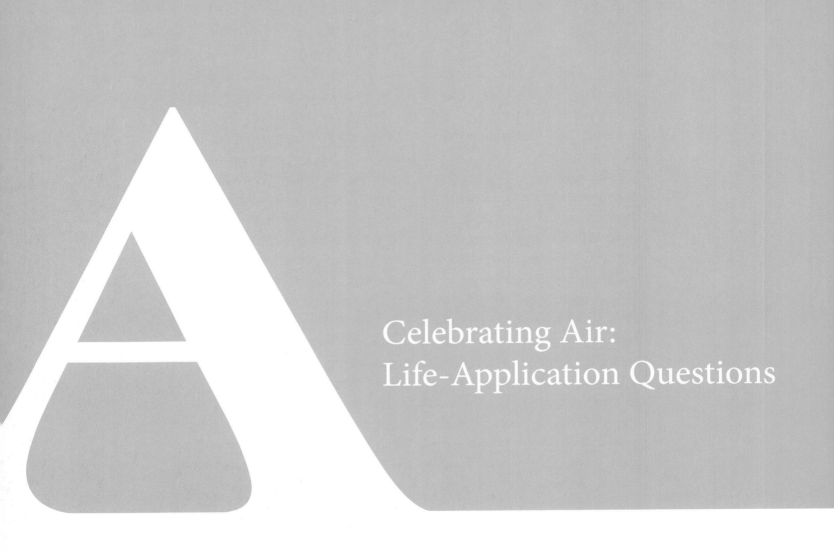

Celebrating Air: Life-Application Questions

Take the time to consider these questions and apply what you are learning to your life.

1 What comes to mind when I consider the wonderful way in which carbon dioxide is continuously removed from the air and oxygen is produced to sustain my life? What is my response to my Creator as I consider the finely tuned mechanism that causes me to breathe at the rate and depth that supply me with a sufficient amount of oxygen? How can I praise and thank Him for this wonderful gift, in both words and actions?

Does the frequent use of vehicles and the amount
of energy sources we use make a difference?

2 How can I ensure that I am making full use of the 3,500 cubic centimeters of air space in my lungs that doesn't get used when I'm doing
quiet breathing? What is "diaphragmatic breathing"? How can I exercise in
a way that forces extra breathing?

GROUP DISCUSSION

3 On his way to work each morning, Samuel passes a street corner
where day laborers wait for someone to give them employment. He
noticed that most of the men smoke or chew tobacco. In what ways could
he help them to recognize the health dangers of tobacco? Would organizing
smoking-cessation programs at his church and inviting them to attend be
beneficial? What effect would distributing brochures or pamphlets on the
dangers of smoking have?

4 Julia yawns a lot after sitting for a long time. Could it be that she
is not breathing well because she's too sedentary? What improvements could she make to her posture while sitting and walking? How much
would one have to move around every half hour to help?

5 What choices can we make that will help reduce global air pollution?
Does the frequent use of vehicles and the amount of electricity and
other energy sources we use make a difference? Are there forums in which
we can participate to advocate for cleaner air, such as the prevention of
smoking in public places? Which trees or shrubs contribute to the cleaning of
the air? What about the option of planting trees on personal property or in
public parks and other community areas?

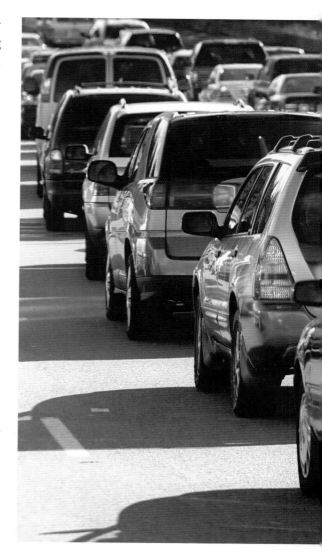

T

Celebrating
Temperance

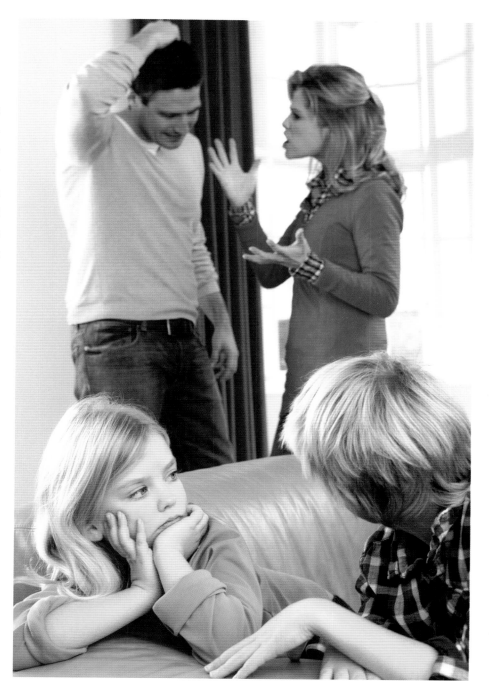

It was a scene of heartrending pain and despondency—children crying as the domestic upheaval they were enduring threatened their comfort zone and emotional security; a frustrated mother, obviously emotional and angry. "This is the last straw!" the mother said to herself. "We can't take it anymore!" Joe, the alcoholic father and husband, had lost yet another job.

A pleasant, soft-spoken man, Joe generally was a kind father and considerate husband—except when under the influence of alcohol. He also was a keen and able sportsman, well liked and welcomed into the sporting circles of his town. He always could be counted on to participate in the celebrations at the clubhouse or pub after a golf game or other sporting event. As his addiction to alcohol cost him one job after another, however, he lost not only his financial security but also the many friends with whom he played, drank, and fraternized during the "better" times.

Joe had a problem not only with alcohol; he also smoked cigarettes. Not

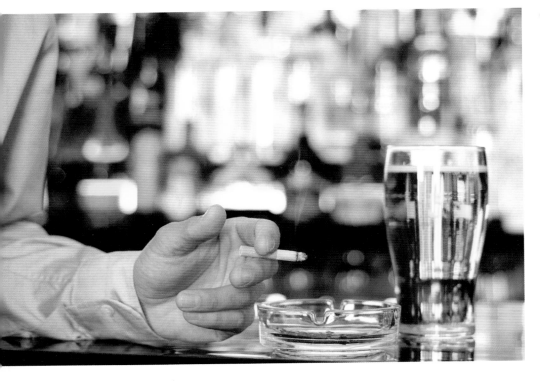

even the diagnosis of cancer of the larynx motivated him to stop smoking for more than a few months. Life-threatening diagnoses such as heart attack and cancer often lead to only short-term lifestyle changes. The sobering reality is that something more is needed to effect meaningful and long-term changes in our established behavior. Joe's sad story bears witness to this pattern, described best in his own words during his numerous but short-lived periods of recovery: "I can control tobacco and alcohol; they are not my master!" The sad reality is that they were his master, and Joe was, in fact, their slave.

Joe's difficulties as a result of his love affair with alcohol affected many others, especially those in his family. Two of his four children also became alcoholics.

THE MEANING OF "TEMPERANCE"

"Temperance" means different things to different people. For some it brings to mind the times of prohibition (when alcohol was legally banned); for others, it relates to childhood and youth instruction on the importance of abstaining from alcohol, tobacco, and recreational drugs. In many cultures and communities "temperance" has become a forgotten (even anachronis-

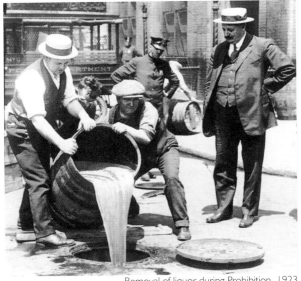

Removal of liquor during Prohibition, 1923

tic) word—a term from the past. So does it still apply to our lives today?

Webster's Dictionary defines "temperance" as "moderation in action, thought, or feeling, or moderation or abstinence from intoxicating drink." This definition includes aspects of behavior and attitude, and specifies that alcoholic beverages be avoided. Is this comprehensive enough? To achieve true balance in life, we need to address all aspects of living; balance in all things is needed. A definition that may move us closer to this wholeness in our living is: "True temperance teaches us to dispense entirely with everything hurtful and to use judiciously that which is healthful."[1] This description implies a way of life as opposed to a checklist of certain substances and behaviors, suggesting that in excess even good things may be harmful!

We can benefit from taking personal stock of our own lives and assets, as to whether we are excessive in eating, working, playing, sleeping, or whatever. It's easy to do an inventory on those around us—what others eat, drink, weigh, drive, wear, and so forth. In some societies conspicuous consumption is obvious, and we have no difficulty identifying it. It's more difficult to analyze our personal attitudes and behaviors to determine whether our own lives are in balance.

What makes matters more complex is that many regard certain destructive habits and lifestyle choices as desirable and even beneficial. Tobacco and alcohol are legal and freely available with very few restrictions. As a result, they've become entwined in cultures and societies worldwide despite the fact that they are the leading and third-leading causes, respectively, of preventable death! The seduction of advertising as well as the stranglehold of commerce have much to do with this tragic situation, but in reality our personal choices play an important role.

One component of being able to make wise choices is the accessibility of information, so let's look at some of the information available.

ALCOHOL CONSUMPTION AND GLOBAL HEALTH

Alcohol consumption varies widely between countries, depending on cultural traditions. There also is a discrepancy between developed and emerging economies. Alcohol, like tobacco, is being exported to developing countries, adding huge burdens to already inadequate health systems. According to the "Global Status Report on Alcohol and Health" released by the World Health Organization (WHO) in Geneva, February 2011:[2]

> True temperance teaches us to dispense entirely with everything hurtful and to use judiciously that which is healthful.
>
> *Patriarchs and Prophets,* p. 562

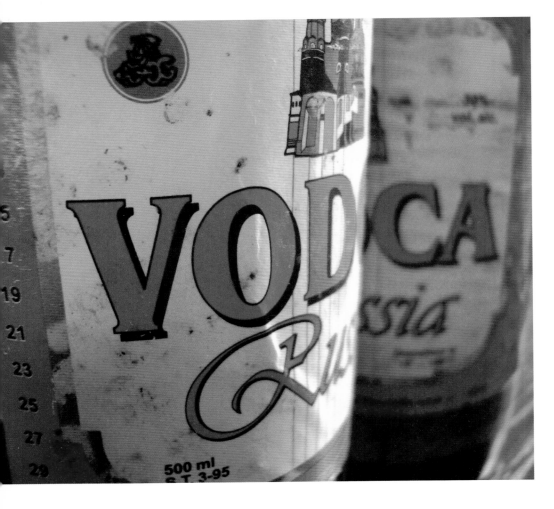

■ Approximately 2.5 million people die from alcohol-related causes each year.

■ Fifty-five percent of adults have consumed alcohol.

■ Four percent of all deaths are related to alcohol through injuries, cancer, cardiovascular diseases, and liver cirrhosis.

■ Globally, 6.2 percent of male deaths are related to alcohol, and 1.1 percent of female deaths.

■ One in five men in the Russian Federation and neighboring countries dies from alcohol-related causes.

The pattern of alcohol consumption is changing, as mentioned previously. Figures for 2001-2005 released by the WHO[3] revealed that worldwide, 6.13 liters of pure alcohol were consumed per year, per person aged 15 years or older. This amount appeared to be stable in the Americas and the European, East-

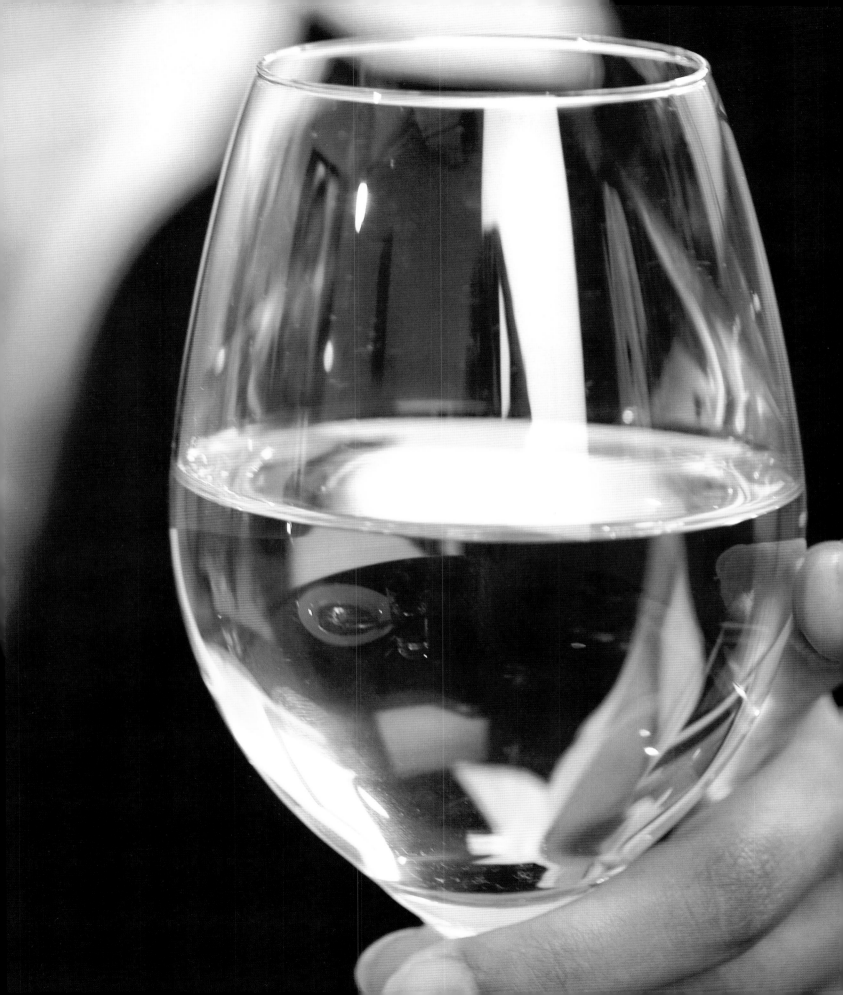

ern Mediterranean, and Western Pacific regions; however, marked increases were noted in Africa and Southeast Asia. Health risk increases even more when binge drinking occurs; in other words, when people drink to get drunk. Binge drinking may be defined differently in various regions of the world: in the United States more than five consecutive drinks for a male and more than four for a female; in Australia more than four drinks on a single occasion. Binge drinking is increasing in many parts of the world, mainly among youth, but all age groups are affected.[4]

A recent book on research and public policy states that "alcohol is a risk factor for a wide range of health conditions and social problems . . . accounting for approximately 4 percent of deaths worldwide and 4.6 percent of the global burden of disease, placing it alongside tobacco as one of the leading preventable causes of death and disability."[5]

Alcohol is no ordinary commodity and is dangerous.

RISKS OF ALCOHOL ADDICTION

Alcohol is a known addictive substance. The likelihood of becoming an alcoholic (euphemistically termed "problem drinker") depends on numerous factors. The chance of alcoholism developing over a lifetime is 13 percent (13 people of every 100 who drink alcohol). If there is a first-degree relative (father, mother, uncle, aunt, grandparent) who suffered from alcohol dependence, this percentage doubles. If experimentation with alcohol begins under the age of 14 years, the percentage chance of dependence increases to 40 percent-plus![6] This demonstrates the importance of alcohol education from an early age and the fostering of relationships and connectedness between responsible adults and youth. Social support develops resilience, enabling youth to cope with difficult decisions and choices despite peer pressure. An additional and vital layer of protection for both young and old is a connection to

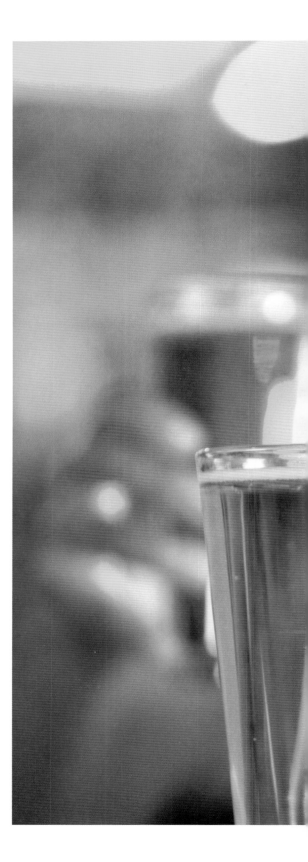

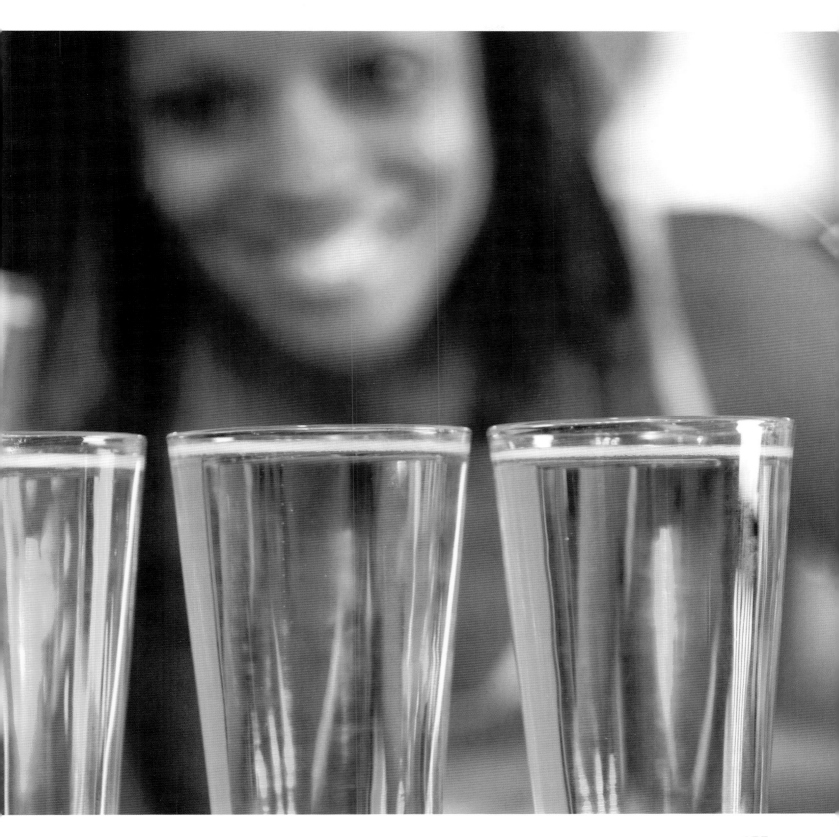

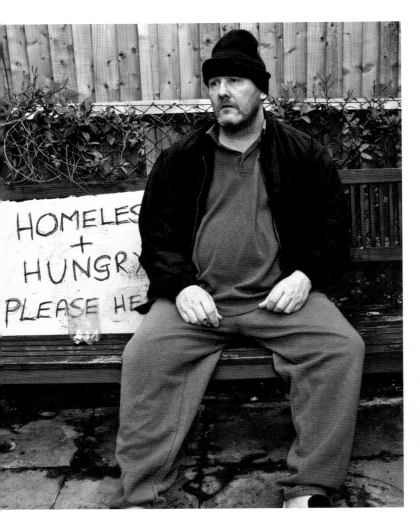

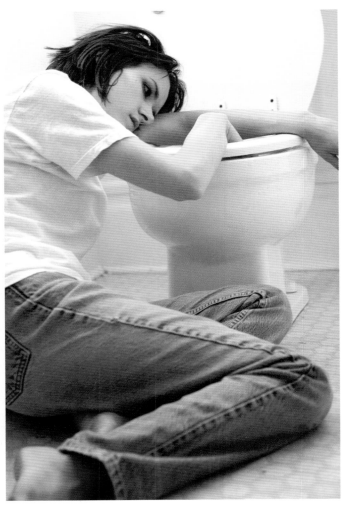

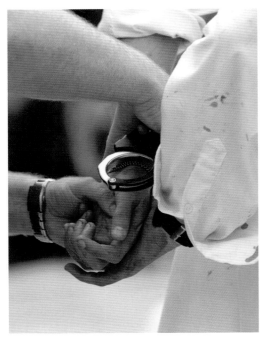

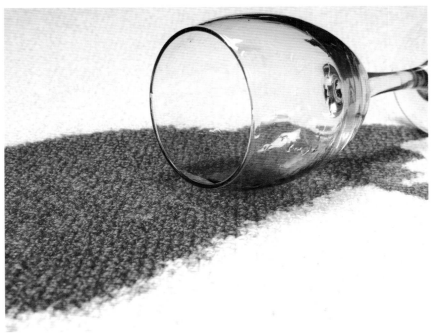

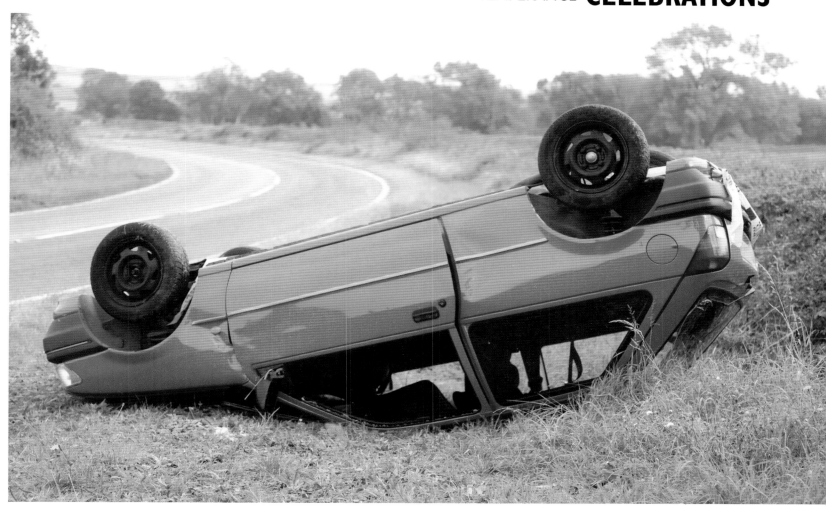

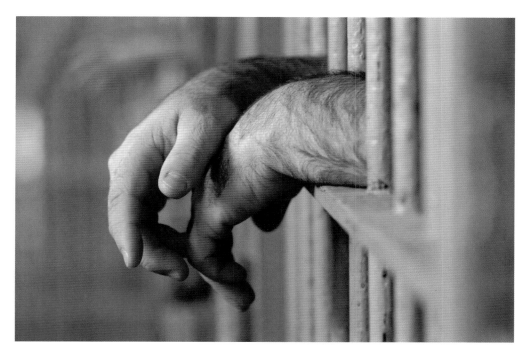

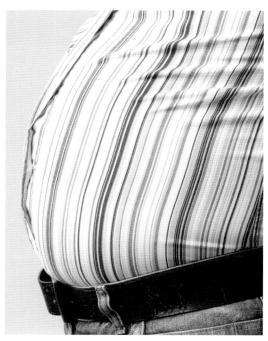

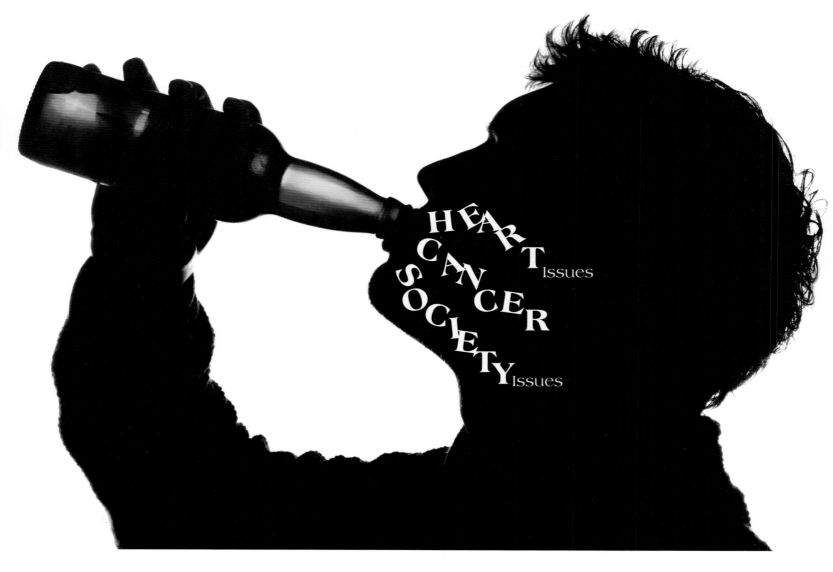

HEART Issues
CANCER
SOCIETY Issues

a set of values, such as the principles of the Bible and walking with the risen Savior.

ALCOHOL AND CANCER

Cancer is one of the leading causes of death globally. An interesting example of the relationship between drinking alcohol and cancer comes from the European Union (EU), where cancer is the second most common cause of death, with 2.5 million cancer deaths per year. It's estimated that 10 percent of cancers in men and 3 percent of cancers in women can be attributed directly to alcohol use. It's further estimated that 30 percent of cancers in the EU could be prevented through more healthful lifestyle choices. The 2010 Eurobarometer Report found, however, that one in five European citizens does not believe that there's a connection between alcohol and cancer; one in ten is totally ignorant that alcohol consumption can cause cancer.[7] Sadly, being ignorant does not spare us the consequences.

Robust evidence links alcohol as a cause of breast cancer in women and colon cancer in both men and women. These findings have been summarized and reported in the World Cancer Research Fund's comprehensive reports in 2007 and 2011.[8] The point strongly emphasized in these and many other scientific reports is that there is no safe limit/

dose of alcohol that can be recommended to avoid its carcinogenic effect. This raises serious doubts about any recommendation that alcohol be used for health benefits, even cardiac, because the associated side effects are real and dangerous.

ALCOHOL AND SOCIETY

It is well known that alcohol use is associated (often causally) with accidents of all kinds, such as road fatalities, as well as domestic violence, murder, rape, and other criminal activities. In 2010 Professor David Nutt and coresearchers published an analysis in the prestigious *The Lancet* medical journal showing that in the United Kingdom alcohol overall is more harmful than heroin and crack cocaine. This is because the researchers focused on the effect the drugs/toxins had not only on the user but others as well (family, community,

and society). Heroin, crack cocaine, and methamphetamine were the most harmful drugs to individuals.[9]

Alcohol is also the leading cause of preventable mental retardation in the world. This is because alcohol readily crosses the placenta and damages the developing brain of the unborn baby. Again, there is no safe level of alcohol consumption during pregnancy.[10]

ALCOHOL AND HEART HEALTH

For the past 30 years alcohol has been promoted as "heart healthy" and protective against coronary artery disease. Much has been written in the popular and scientific literature on the subject. None of the scientific studies have been controlled, randomized, prospective analyses, which makes them even more subject to what are known as "confounders." Confounders are factors that make interpretation of the results of the data being analyzed more difficult and also may result in erroneous conclusions. Naimi and

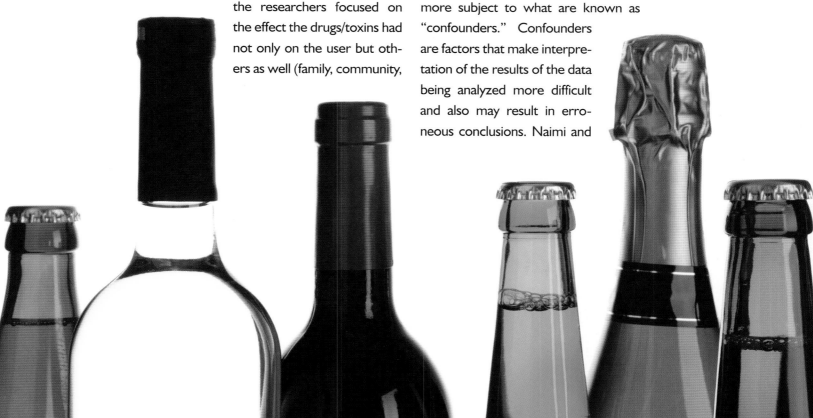

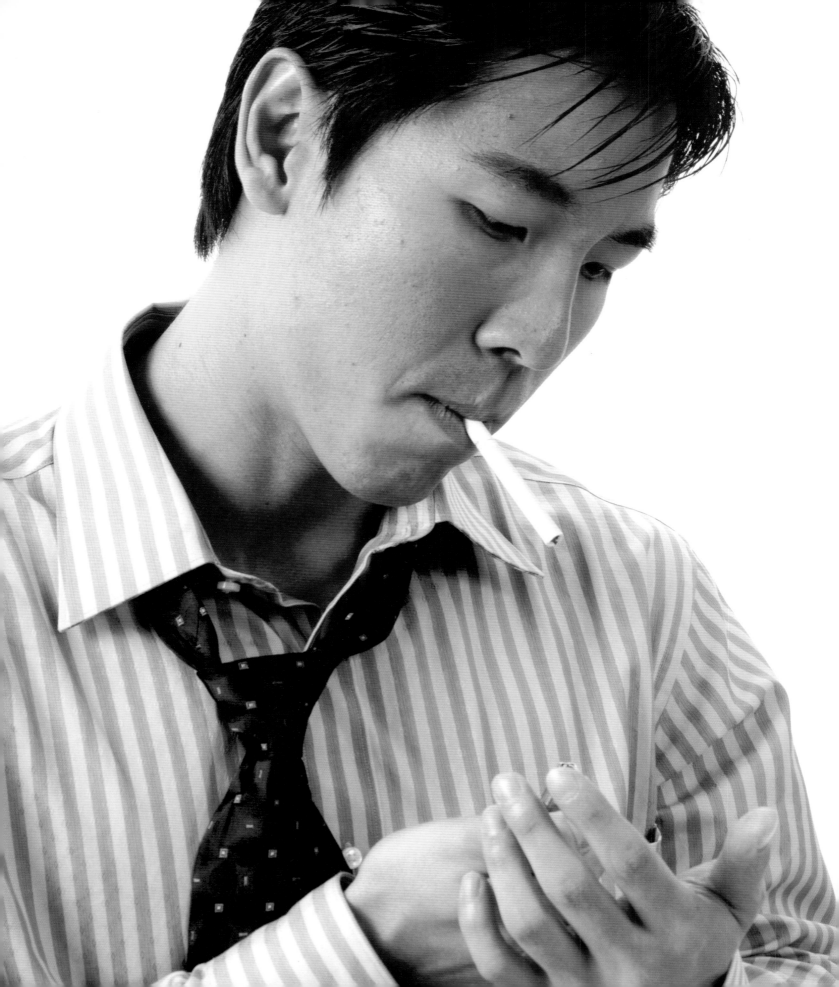

other researchers concluded in 2005 that some or all of the apparent cardiac protective effect of moderate drinking may be the result of these confounders.[11] Other studies have sounded caution and noted that the nondrinkers included in many of the studies had more risk factors for heart disease, were less well-educated, had less access to health care and insurance, and were from poorer socioeconomic groups. Some included in the nondrinking group had been drinkers prior to the studies being done and had stopped drinking for health reasons.[12] A recent paper by Dr. Boris Hansel adds weight to the view that the real explanation of positive cardiac outcomes in moderate drinkers is not that alcohol is protective, but that the average health status and healthful lifestyle in other behaviors, such as exercise and diet, are better than that of nondrinkers.[13]

In summary, taking into account the significant health risks related to alcohol use, it doesn't make sense to promote its use for heart health, especially when there are proven and safe interventions for heart-disease prevention such as daily exercise and a healthful diet.

KILLER TOBACCO

There is another lethal and freely available poison that is marketed in various forms—tobacco. It's smoked, chewed, inhaled, and passed through water; all forms, however, are harmful and place the user at significant risk of disease and even death. It's surprising that tobacco is so popular when you consider that it kills up to half its users!

◼ Tobacco kills nearly 6 million people each year. Of this number more than 5 million are users and ex-users, and more than 600,000 are nonsmokers exposed to secondhand smoke. Without urgent intervention the annual death toll could rise to some 8 million by 2030.

◼ Nearly 80 percent of the world's 1 billion smokers live in low- and middle-income countries.

◼ Consumption of tobacco products is increasing globally.

◼ Approximately 1 person dies every 6 seconds as a result of tobacco-related causes.

◼ Up to half of current users will eventually die of a tobacco-related disease.

Tobacco is a gradual killer. There's a lag of several years between initiation of tobacco use and when the user's health suffers. It's one of the most significant public health threats the world has ever faced, killing not only the user but often negatively impacting the health of, or even killing, those who are exposed to secondhand tobacco smoke.

Secondhand smoke (SHS) by definition is the smoke that fills restaurants, offices, homes, and any enclosed space in which tobacco products including cigarettes, cigars, pipes, bidis, and water pipes (shisha) are burned. There is no safe level of exposure to secondhand smoke. It's a proven cause of cardiovascular and respiratory disease in adults, including lung cancer and coronary heart disease. SHS also is associated with Sudden Infant Death Syndrome (SIDS) and causes low birth weight in pregnant women. Children exposed to

SHS have an increased incidence of upper- and lower-respiratory infections.

All these complications, both from primary inhalation of tobacco smoke and SHS exposure, result from the many toxins, chemicals, and nicotine in tobacco smoke. There are more than 2,000 chemicals in tobacco smoke; at least 250 of these are known to be harmful, and more than 50 are known carcinogens (initiate cancer).

Tobacco is a "gateway drug."[14] This means that people who are exposed to tobacco are on the threshold of using and becoming addicted to other drugs, such as marijuana, methamphetamine, cocaine, and heroin. This is par-ticularly significant when considering tobacco use by young people, which is becoming more common in many parts of the world. The age of debut is getting younger, as well. Long-term addiction to tobacco is also more likely when individuals initiate smoking at a young age.

In summary, both alcohol and tobacco are extremely dangerous substances. Scientific evidence and public health statistics show them to be leading killers in the world today. Of course, it's left to one's personal choices as to whether to indulge, and this is where temper-ance has such a wise safeguard: avoid all things harmful! The facts surely speak for themselves.

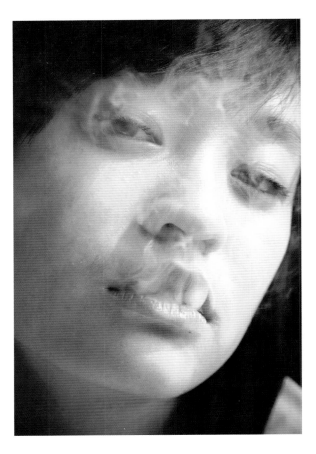

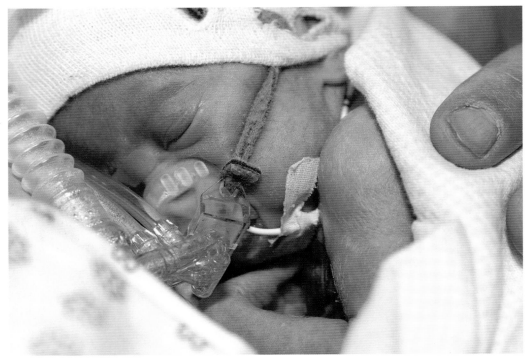

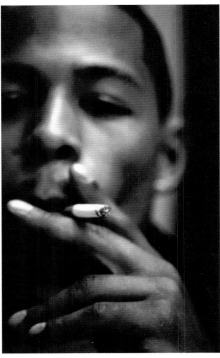

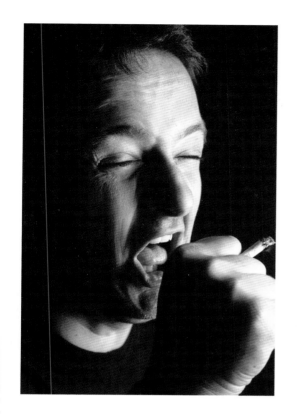

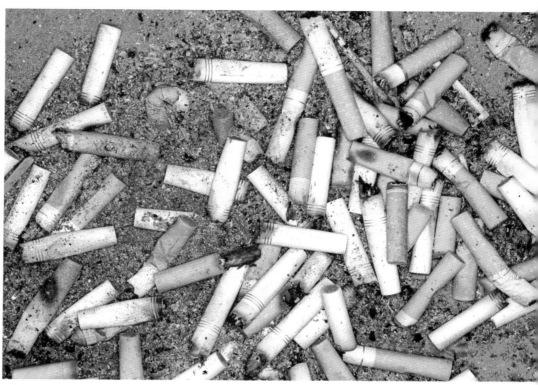

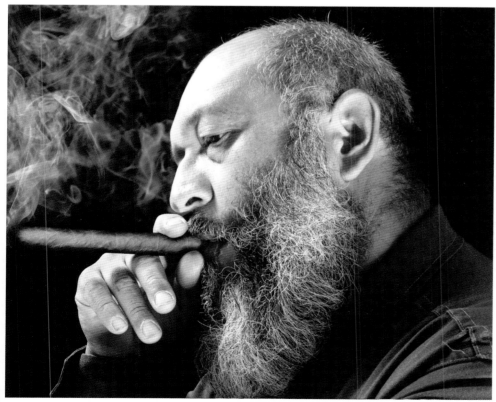

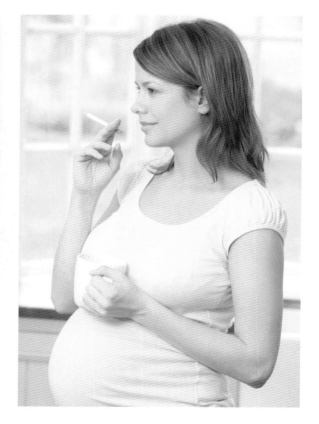

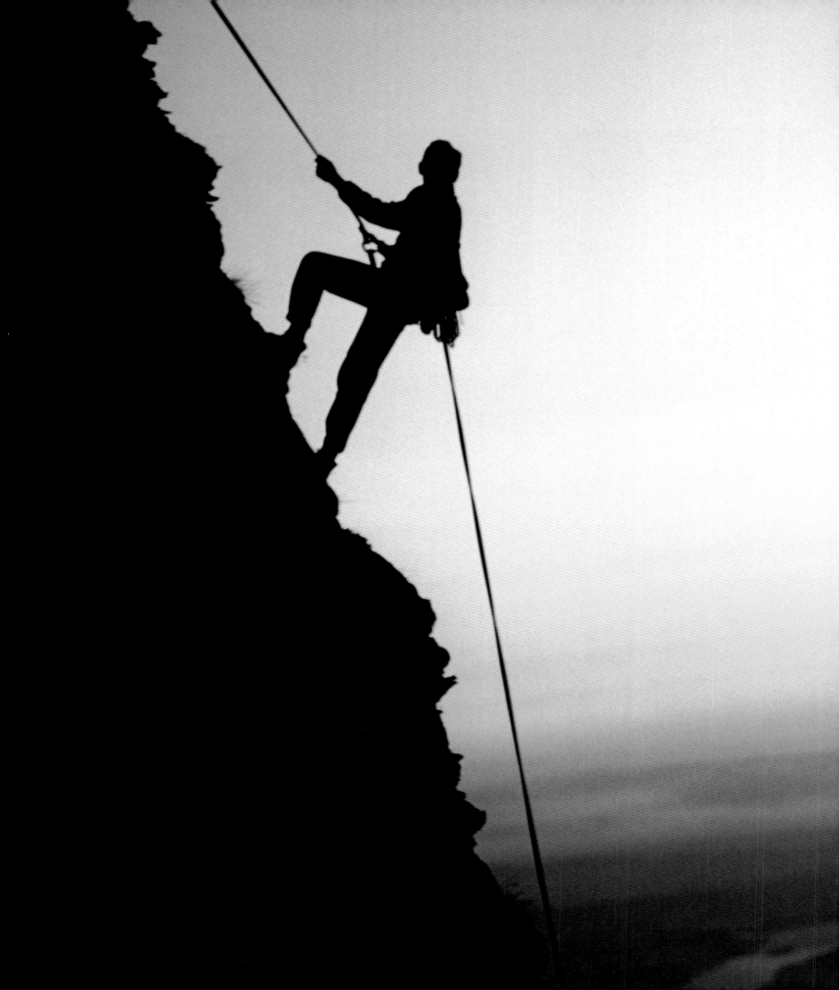

I can do everything through him
who gives me strength. Phil. 4:13. NIV

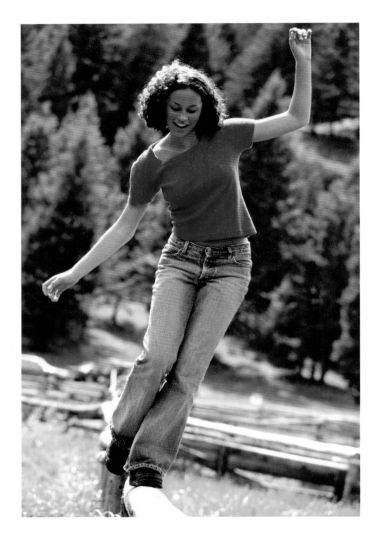

TRUE BALANCE IN LIVING

Joe's story reveals the consequences of failing to avoid all things harmful. As we take stock of our own lives there may be areas in which we lack balance such as sleeping too little, working too hard, not exercising enough (or maybe overdoing it), eating too much, and the list goes on. We may even abuse social media or the availability of the Internet with its seductive and misleading pornography menus. These forms of technology are good in themselves but potentially addictive when not used judiciously. Even the most strong-willed among us is unable to achieve true balance in all things without a strong reliance on the power of our gracious and Almighty God, who not only made us but is able to sustain us and strengthen our will and ability to make wise choices.

Remember Paul's counsel in Scripture: "Whether you eat or drink or whatever you do, do it all for the glory of God" (1 Cor. 10:31, NIV). Realizing that this is a very tall order, Paul fortunately adds the secret of power and success: "I can do everything through him who gives me strength" (Phil. 4:13, NIV).

It's encouraging to remember that help is never far away. "[God] is not far from each one of us. For in him we live and move and have our being" (Acts 17:27, 28, NIV). Our gracious heavenly Father stands ready to guide our choices, ensuring a sustained and successful true balance in life. This calls for celebration!

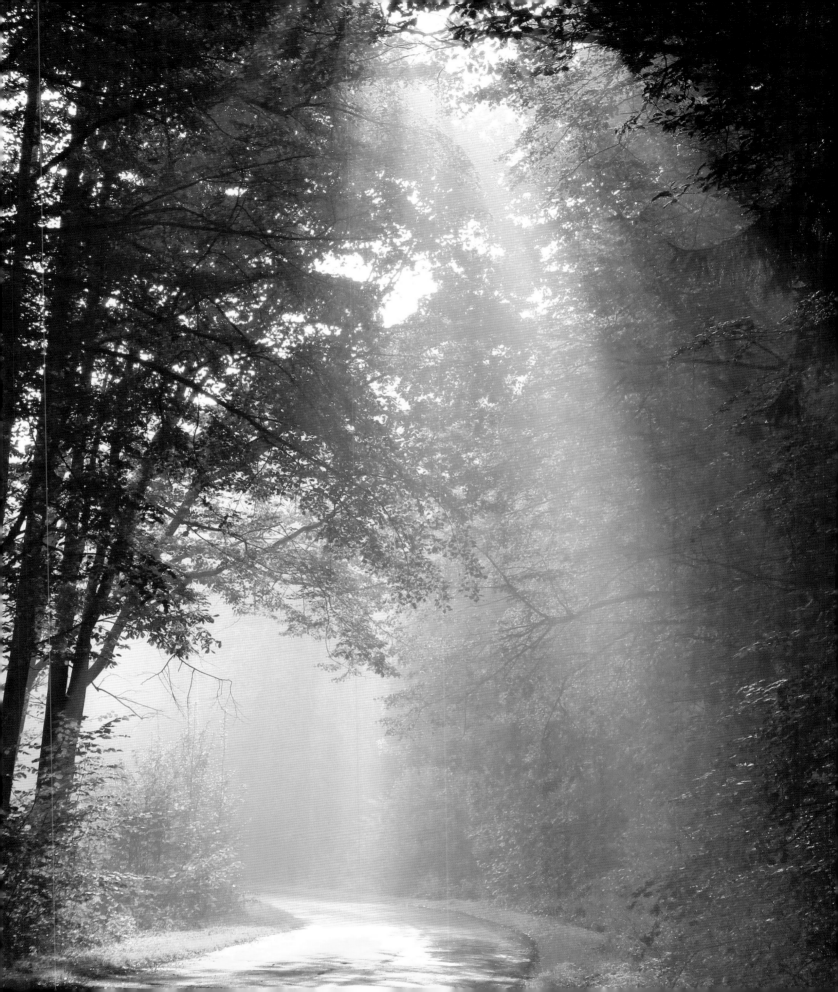

Celebrating Temperance: Life-Application Questions

Take the time to consider these questions and apply what you are learning to your life.

1 Have I been influenced by articles that purport that drinking a little alcohol is beneficial to the cardiac system? What other negative consequences of alcohol use support these reports? If I were to drink only socially, what are my chances of becoming addicted? Do I have a first-degree relative who has suffered from alcohol dependence? If so, how would that affect the risk I would be taking?

How do I know if I am working too much, sleeping too little, eating too much, or exercising too little?

2 What things in my life are out of control, unbalanced, or used injudiciously? How do I know if I am working too much, sleeping too little, eating too much, or exercising too little? How do I make judicious use of my free time? Am I spending too much time with electronic media and too little time cultivating good relationships with my Savior and people close to me? Do I set aside time for service to those less fortunate? When I realize the need for change, do I remember the One who can give me the strength I need? Do I ask for that enabling power?

GROUP DISCUSSION

3 A group of boys and girls from a local church school attended a party at which binge drinking occurred. Unfortunately, they found the alcohol in the church member's home. If asked to give regular talks at the school on the dangers associated with alcohol, which of the facts in this story should be emphasized? Is our example of temperance one they should follow?

4 How can we reduce the chances of children and youth in our homes, churches, or communities being pressured by their peers into experimenting with tobacco, alcohol, or other drugs? Would it make a difference to take time to know their names and greet and interact with them? Are we examples that they would want to emulate?

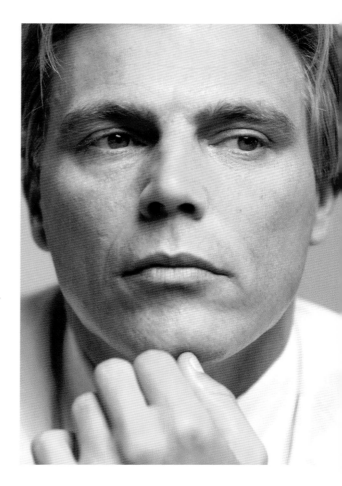

Celebrating Integrity

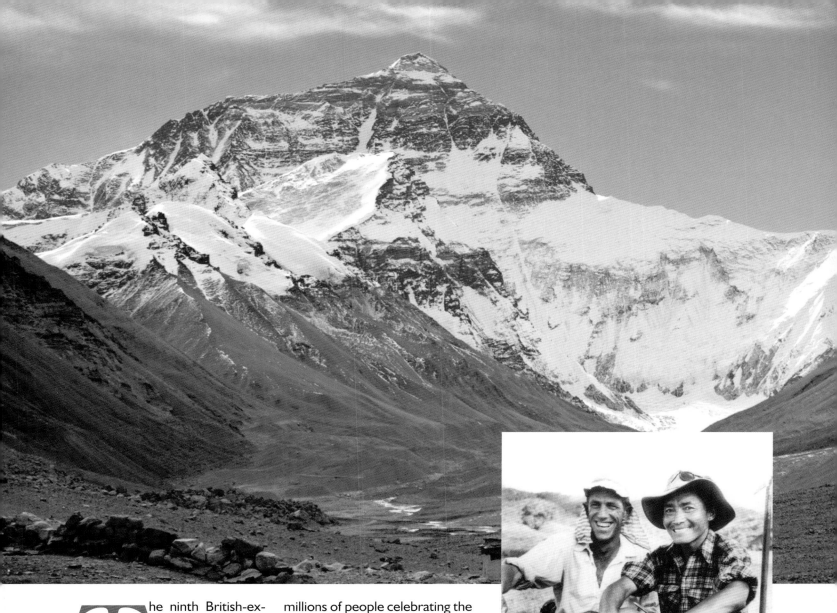

Edmund Hillary and Tensing Norgay, 1953

The ninth British-expedition attempt to scale the height of Everest, the world's highest mountain, took place in May 1953. Led by John Hunt, the climbers were paired into teams, and Tom Bourdillon and his partner, Charles Evans, came to within 300 feet of the peak. Oxygen problems forced their return to camp, but by creating a trail and leaving behind equipment, they facilitated the successful ascent by Edmund Hillary and Tensing Norgay. For the millions of people celebrating the coronation of Queen Elizabeth II on June 2, 1953, this news added a frenzy of exhilaration to the already excited populace.

For several years this first ascent of Everest was labeled a "team effort," with "we reached the top together" being the news release. A few years later, however, Tensing said that "only the truth is good enough for Everest," and then indicated that Hillary had put his foot on the peak first. Such honesty speaks to the integrity of Tensing Norgay.

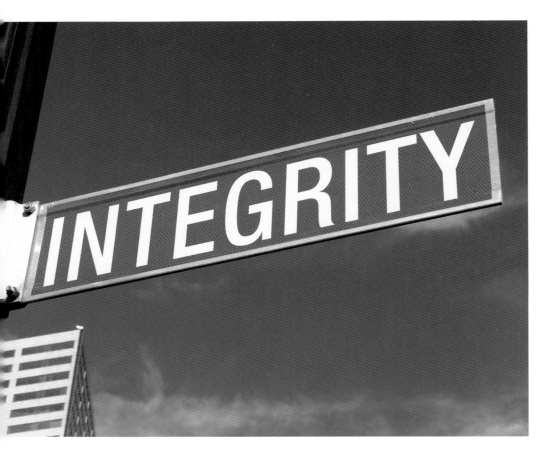

Integrity means there is a commitment to the principles espoused as being correct.

Integrity—as strange as it may seem—is also an essential factor in the prescription for the vital and exuberant celebration of health. It's a motivational ingredient that is very much at work in the implementation of health practices.

The distinction between integrity and simple honesty at times may be unclear. Integrity is a concordance in the life between theory and practice. It's the transparency and trustworthiness that should characterize our every action. When there is a difference between what we say and what we do, we demonstrate a need for integrity.

On the Yahoo Web site forum "Yahoo Answers," questions were raised on the meaning of honesty and integrity and the difference between the two. Among the answers were these two:

"Honesty means that whatever you've done—good or bad—you speak the truth about it. In other words, you don't lie."

"Integrity means that you adhere to a moral conviction or code of honor that won't allow you to do certain things that you feel would debase you."

While not dictionary definitions, these Yahoo answers illustrate the role integrity plays in determining our actions. Honesty may lead to confession or admission of guilt, but it may not be sufficient to influence behavior. Integrity means there is a commitment to the principles espoused as being correct.

While still a young South African lawyer, Mahatma Gandhi committed to the cause of justice and by example taught others the power and influence of integrity. George Ludwig recounts the following story:

"A mother once brought her child to him, asking him to tell the young boy not to eat sugar because it was not good for his diet or his developing teeth. Gandhi replied, 'I cannot tell him that. But you may bring him back in a month.'

"The mother was angry as Gandhi moved on, brushing her aside. She had traveled some distance and had expected the mighty leader to support her parenting. She had little recourse, so she left for her home. One month later she returned, not knowing what to expect.

"The great Gandhi took the small child's hands into his own, knelt down before him, and tenderly communicated, 'Do not eat sugar, my child. It is not good for you.' Then he embraced him and returned the boy to his mother. The mother, grateful but perplexed, queried, 'Why didn't you say that a month ago?'

"'Well,' said Gandhi, 'a month ago I was still eating sugar.'"[1]

What power in example! What power in integrity!

INTEGRITY AND PUBLIC HEALTH

Integrity can influence both an individual's as well as a community's health, because it calls for both loyalty and commitment to honest codes of belief and behavior.

In dealing with community health it's essential to recognize the meaning of even subtle aspects of values, morality, ethics, and beliefs. In fact, the Public Health Leadership Society in 2002 published "Principles of the Ethical Practice of Public Health," a document representing a consensus on a code of behavior for public health protagonists.[2] We will touch on only a few of the 12 principles the document addressed.

The first of these opinions deals with an individual's health and states: "Humans have a right to the resources necessary for health."

This is an affirmation of article 25 of the "United Nations' Universal Declaration of Human Rights." Such

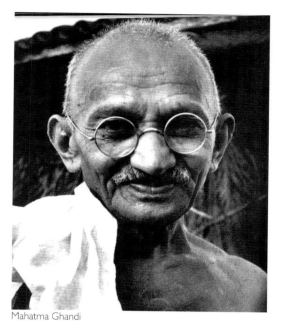
Mahatma Ghandi

What power in example! What power in integrity!

belief will influence many aspects of how we live and model health principles, and will also provide a basis for health education. It has a major impact on ethical behavior and will highlight the degree of integrity with which we function as a society regarding health.

Focusing on our community, the second belief and value states: "Humans are inherently social and interdependent."

As the document points out, "The rightful concern for the physical individuality of humans and one's right to make decisions for oneself must be balanced against the fact that each person's actions affect other people."

Acceptance of this belief raises questions of integrity in how we relate to issues such as smoking and immunization and their effect on public health. Immunization programs, for example, may challenge our integrity as we consider our responsibility to the group when it comes to accepting or refusing immunization. We should keep in mind factors such as recent outbreaks of measles and their resultant morbidity and mortality, which have been traced to pockets of religious adherents who have declined immunization for their members and children.

This belief also will pose questions about the regulation of the availability of drugs that include prescription medications, alcohol, and substances often used in a so-called "recreational" fashion.

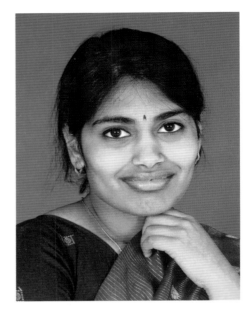

Integrity leads to absolute transparency, open accountability, and is the measure of our reliability. This, in turn, is a very important factor in the area of trust, which undergirds the use and effectiveness of health-care institutions, physicians, and allied health professionals.

The society's 12 principles include the need for collaboration, an important ingredient in effective support of community health. It becomes a matter of integrity to balance personal biases and desires against community needs.

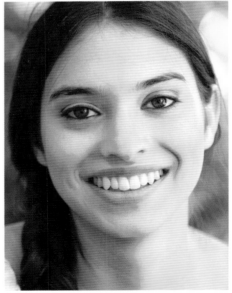

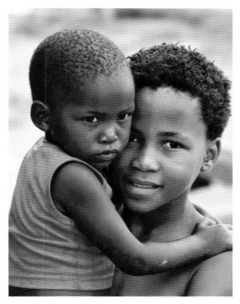
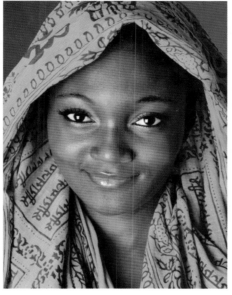
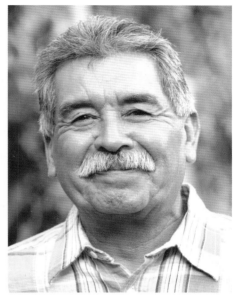
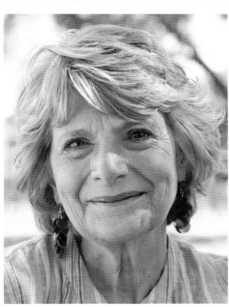
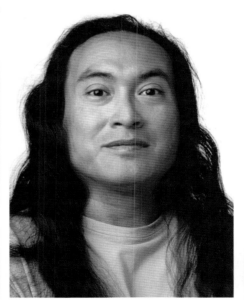
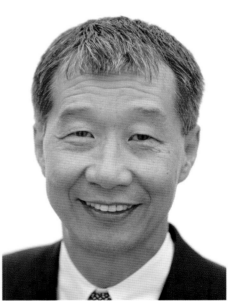

Because "people are dependent upon their physical environment," as stated in the "Principles" document, we have a duty to preserve and sustain the environment. Integrity demands this of us.

Recognizing the value of each individual, we will ensure that all have a voice and are heard in public discourse. Such action may seem to be common courtesy, but sometimes in matters of health, our personal convictions are so keenly felt that we are intolerant of another's opinion and belief. If we claim to believe in the individual's value, we are called by integrity to give opportunity and ear to others' opinions. Integrity demands tolerance of people, even if we disagree with their opinions.

Another value of the "Principles of the Ethical Practice of Public Health" is "Identify and promote the fundamental requirements for health in a community."

Often we substitute individual preferences for community needs, emphasizing the peripheral, borderline, unimportant, or trivial while areas of major impor-tance are ignored. Typical of such personal bias would be an emphasis on avoiding soy products, dairy, certain oils, etc., in situations of famine, drought, poverty, or inequitable availability of a variety of foodstuffs. Integrity will require of us a balance in teaching, practice, and advocacy of certain health practices.

INTEGRITY AND PERSONAL HEALTH

Integrity has personal as well as public health ramifications. It would teach us to recognize our common vulnerability and inherent weaknesses, but also our intrinsic worth and rightful equality as humans with inalienable rights. Such insight influences our belief in our commonality, our kinship in the human family, and our value to society in general. A great deal of mental ill health could be avoided if we possessed sufficient integrity that we would not impose our will on others, nor allow ourselves to be depreciated in our own eyes by the opinions of others.

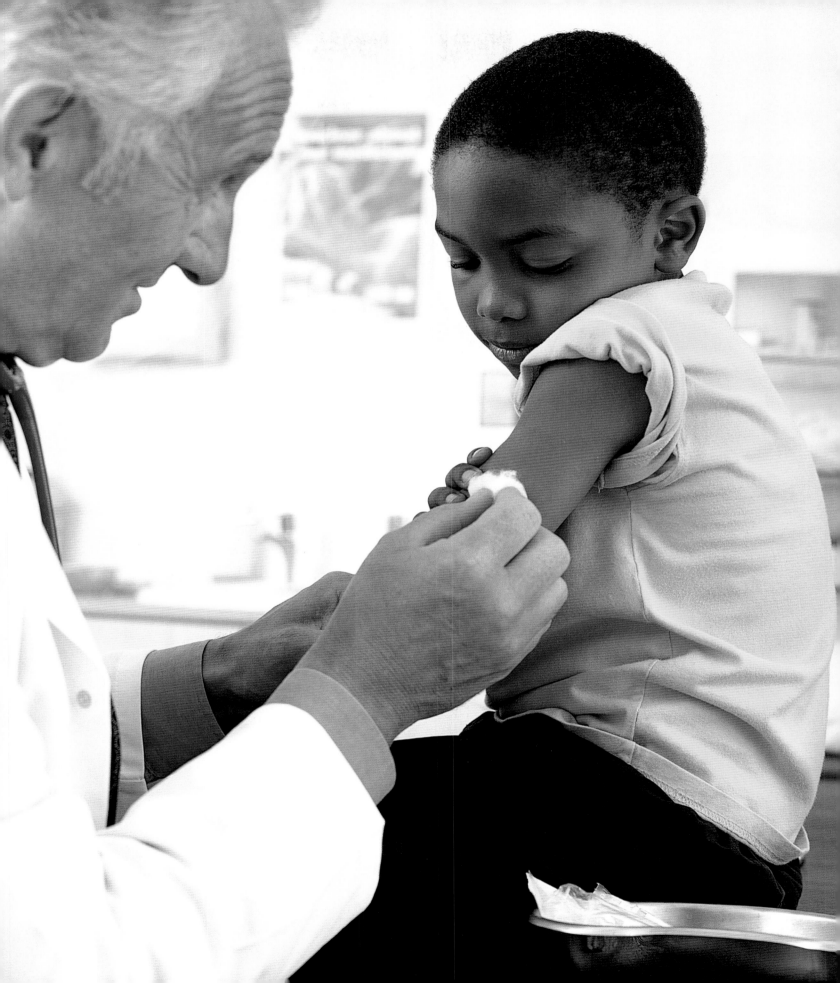

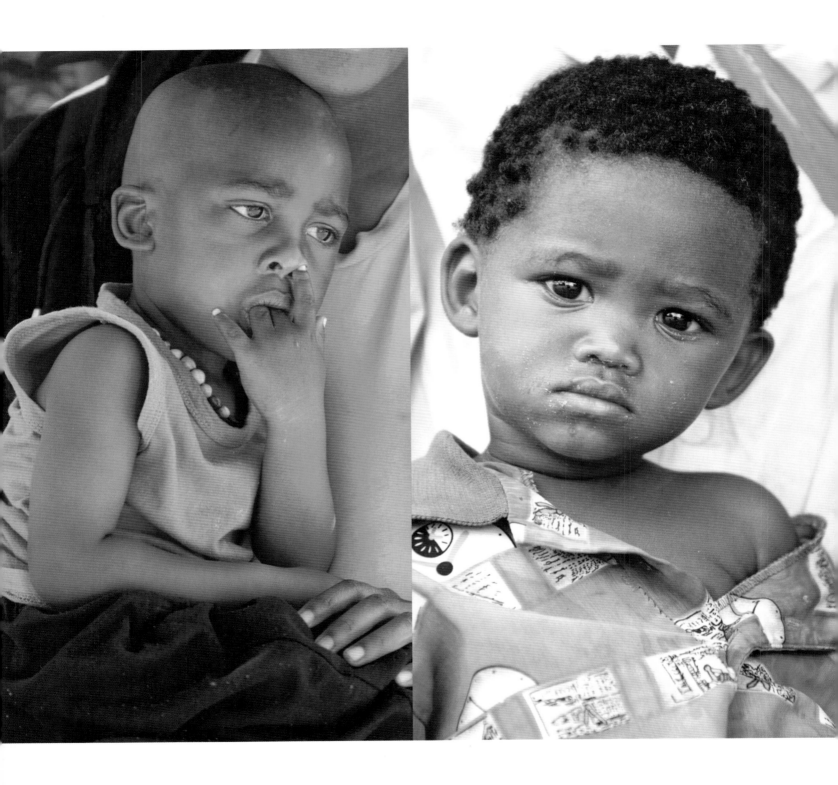

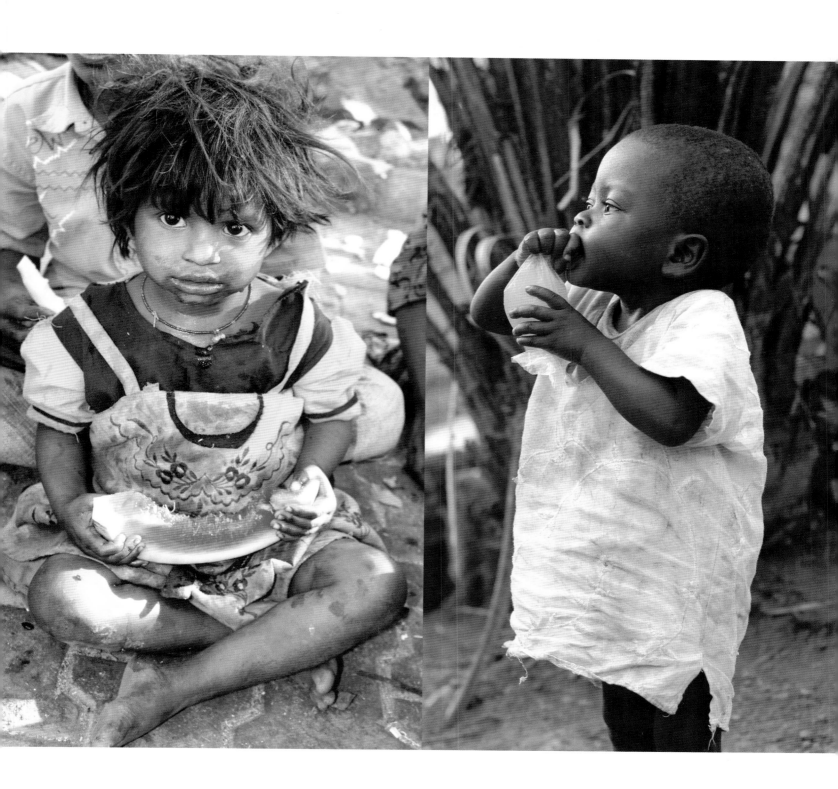

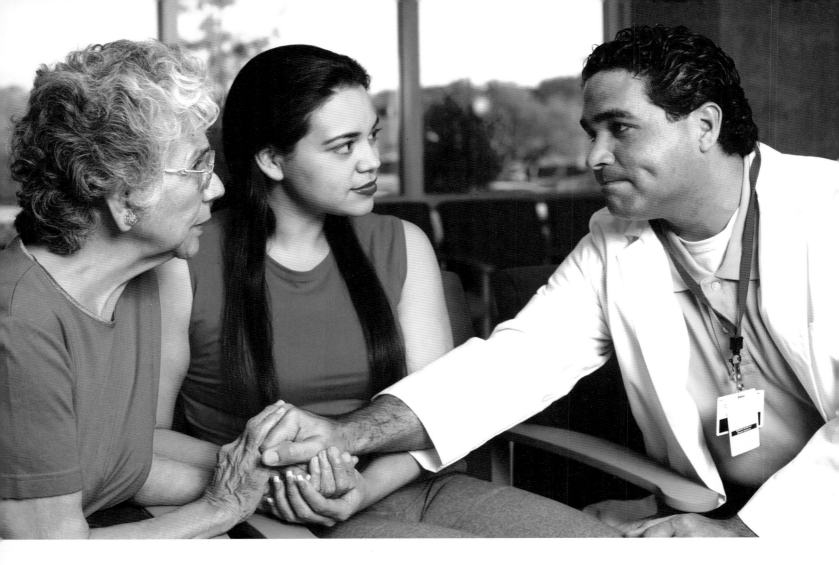

ACT ON PRINCIPLES, NOT OPINIONS

To those whose actions are based on principle, integrity brings motivational insight. Humans are extremely vulnerable to distortions of fact, especially when it comes to personal behaviors.

This is an ancient problem. We are distractible. Michelangelo, perhaps the world's most renowned of artists, wrote, "The world's frivolities have robbed me of the time that I was given for reflecting upon God." Integrity focuses our minds on truth, meaningfulness, value, and reality. When we address issues of health in this way, we'll find that we're dishonest most often with ourselves. The trite, frivolous, faddish, exotic, improbable, and sheer idiotic cease to captivate if we are truly honest. Integrity helps us to examine the evidence and recognize our own biases.

It demands of us high standards and requires us to base our beliefs upon evidence, not fancy. In essence, integrity denies us hypocrisy.

INTEGRITY CAN HELP
US AVOID PROBLEMS

Have you ever wondered how many addicts started down the road to ruin because they ignored the dangers of which they were well aware? Possessing integrity has protected thousands who have declined an offer of drugs, even though fascinated by the potential pleasure.

How many smokers ignored known facts in an effort to "fit in" or appear sophisticated? It's far different to become an addict through ignorance than by deliberately ignoring the truth.

178

When we know that 7 percent of persons taking their first alcoholic drink will become alcoholics, and some 15 percent will have alcohol-related problems such as physical or sexual abuse or be harmed in an accident,[3] shouldn't we question our integrity if we serve such beverages?

Perhaps the most dangerous area regarding integrity is sexual behavior. The media trivializes marital infidelity and encourages sexual irresponsibility in the face of staggering numbers of single-parent children, insecurity, and emotional distress; this raises a question of corporate integrity.

On June 6, 1981, the U.S. Centers for Disease Control (CDC) published the first report of a new syndrome. The report described five young men who had an acquired immune-deficiency syndrome labeled AIDS, for short.[4] Since then, millions upon millions have died, and millions more live with the virus. In Africa, the disease has orphaned more than 15 million children.

HIV/AIDS has raised dozens of questions of corporate integrity regarding such groups as the medical practitioners who declined to treat such patients, the pharmaceutical industry that held patients to excessive ransom, the governments that denied the existence of the disease, and the agencies that controlled blood products and moved so slowly that hundreds became infected.

The disease also challenged individual

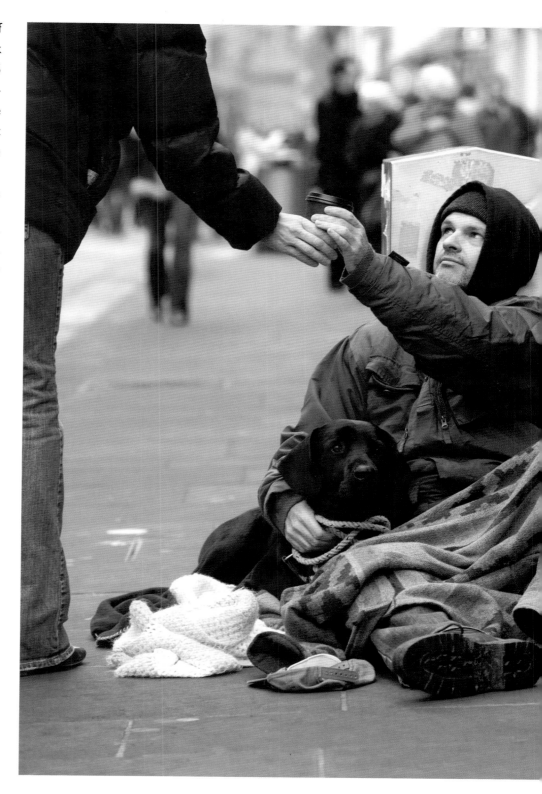

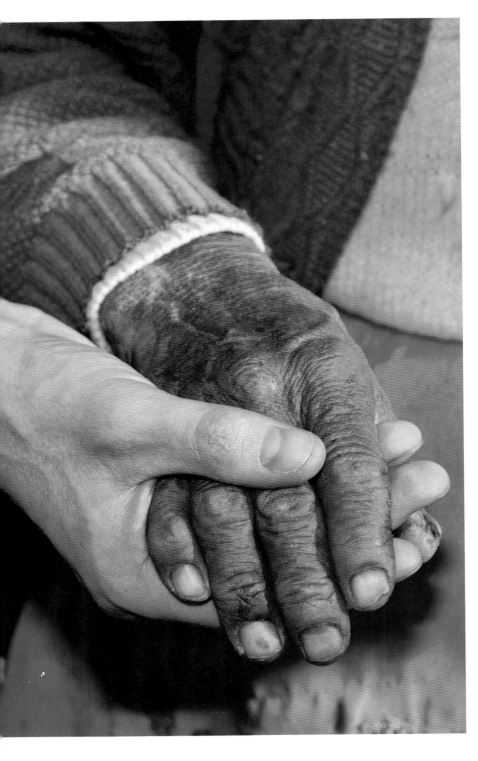

integrity: persons who willfully infected others, partners who denied the other the protection of a condom, and clerics who interfered without sufficient knowledge of the marital interactions of their parishioners. Then seldom addressed is the lack of integrity in promiscuous behavior by single and married individuals.

Integrity impacts many aspects of living. We tend to compartmentalize our behaviors into work, church, social, and intellectual slots, resulting in glaring inconsistencies of integrity when we fail to integrate them. Integrity is the foundation for good mental health, trustworthy interpersonal relationships, and responsible and accountable behavior.

MERCY AND FORGIVENESS

At one time or another everyone has failed to meet the standard of full integrity. Possibly, we have failed so miserably that someone has suffered. We may bear a burden of guilt and remorse.

Forgiveness is not easy for individuals to extend to others, but Jesus Christ described a forgiving God. He lived and died to exemplify grace. All the religions of the world teach that forgiveness is attainable. Some require penance; Jesus Christ requires only contrition.

By the gift of grace God extends mercy and forgiveness. Even here, integrity is essential. We have to be honest enough to admit wrongdoing; it is by such confession that grace permits peace and rest to be attained. If we are to celebrate the completeness of whole-person health, integrity is essential.

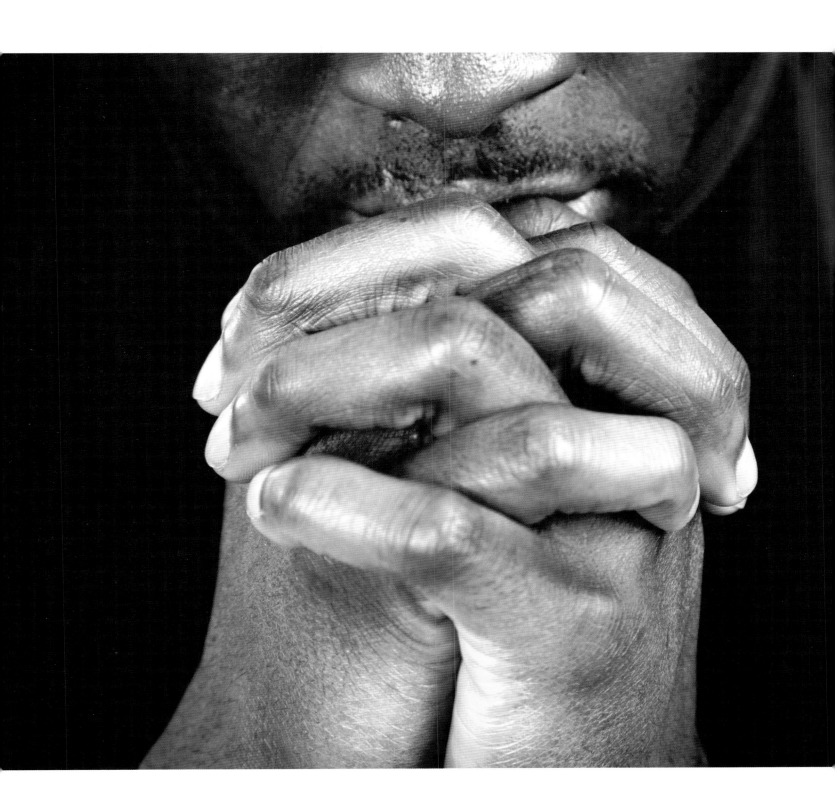

Celebrating Integrity:
Life-Application Questions

Take the time to consider these questions and apply what you are learning to your life.

1 Do I consider myself to be an honest person? What moral values have I adopted that prevent me from doing anything that would conflict with that code of honor? What sources have formed that set of values?

2 What can I do to ensure that others trust what I say to them is in their best interest and not just my way of pushing my own personal beliefs? Am I promoting any health practices, dietary principles, etc., that would be unsuitable for a given situation in which I am not involved? Do I grant others the ability to hold their own opinions, even when I am sure I am right?

3 What personal choices fly in the face of evidence but are comfortable or desirable just because they are what I want to do? What evidence presented in this book have I disregarded because it would be difficult or unpleasant to have to fit certain practices into my lifestyle?

4 Have I violated my code of honor? Do I admit my wrongdoing? What do I do with the guilt I feel because I have not lived up to my values? Do I punish myself by dwelling on my guilt or fall into a cycle of repeating the behavior again and again? Or can I accept the mercy and forgiveness that Jesus freely offers?

GROUP DISCUSSION

5 Along with considering personal health, in what ways can we also take into account the needs of the community and how personal choices could affect others? What choices with respect to personal hygiene, such as hand washing and staying away from contact with others when ill, could positively affect our communities? What practices for personal pleasure may have negative effects on others?

6 A local church health ministries leader regularly presents lectures to the church members in which she advocates a total vegetarian diet. She also favors an organic diet, although she is aware that many of the members cannot afford the higher prices for organic foods. Sometimes, however, she invites others to go with her to an ice cream parlor where she enjoys ice cream as a "special treat." What lifestyle practices do we have that may conflict with what we "preach"? Are we truly "walking the talk"?

What lifestyle practices do I have that may conflict with what I "preach"?

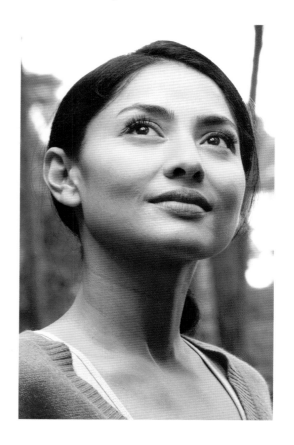

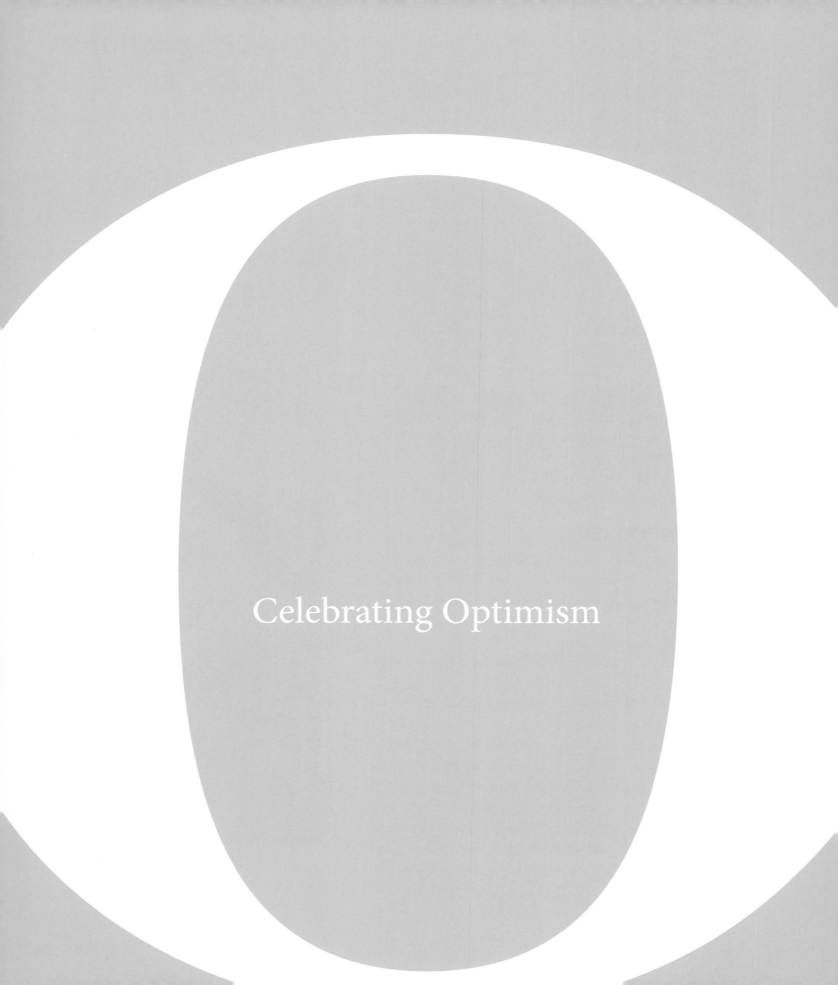

Celebrating Optimism

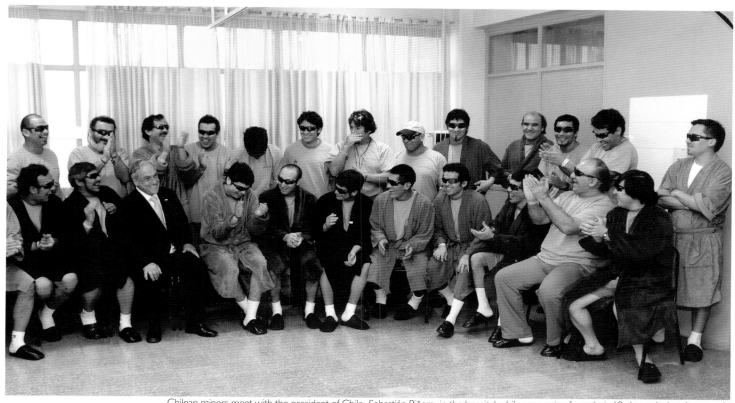

Chilean miners meet with the president of Chile, Sebastián Piñera, in the hospital while recovering from their 69-day ordeal underground.

Suddenly they were unable to see. Thick dust not only blocked the artificial light but irritated and burned their eyes for six hours. It was shortly after lunch when the routine of the day changed—and so has the story of history.

On August 5, 2010, a rockfall in the Chilean Copiapó copper mine trapped 33 miners 2,300 feet underground. Another group of miners that was nearer the entrance of the mine was able to escape, but for the 33 it was another story. Their world had collapsed around them.

Uppermost in their minds was the need to survive and escape. The shift leader, Luis Urzúa, immediately took charge and organized the men into a team that made all their decisions on a democratic basis—the majority votes carried each action and plan.

Ventilation problems forced the men to move out of their 540-square-foot (50-square-meter) emergency shelter into a tunnel. They had access to 1.2 miles (2 kilometers) of galleries in which to move around. Lack of emergency ladders hampered vain attempts to escape through ventilation shafts. Their two- to three-day emer-

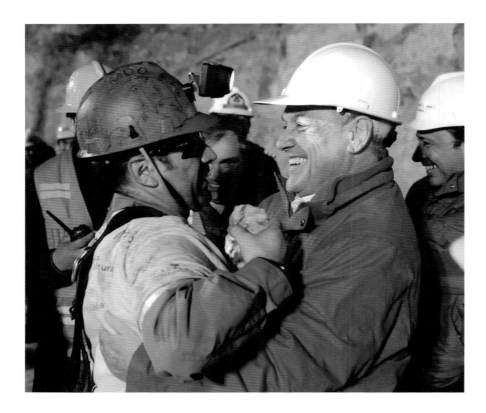

gency supplies were stretched to last two weeks. Careful rationing, strict discipline, social support, and camaraderie all came into play.

Each of the men lost an average of 18 pounds (8 kilograms) in weight. For some, this was an uncomfortable but needed advantage; otherwise they may not have fit into the escape capsules when ultimately found.

On August 22 a drill bored its eighth hole and broke into a shaft close to where the trapped miners were anxiously anticipating rescue. For days the miners had heard the drills and prepared notes to attach to the drill bit. The now famous paper was attached with the words: "We are well in the shelter, the 33." Joy and excitement broke out both above and below ground level; however, there was uncertainty as to how the rescue would be executed and concern that it could take many months to complete.

During this time another interesting phenomenon occurred: a tent city sprang up in the desert near the mine entrance. At first, family and friends slept in cars and waited and prayed. Friends then brought tents and other supplies to help those keeping vigil to survive the hostile desert environment. The settlement was appropriately named Campamento Esperanza (Camp Hope).

Multicultural collaboration, engineering ingenuity, careful planning, and dogged determination led to the miners emerging one by one, safe and

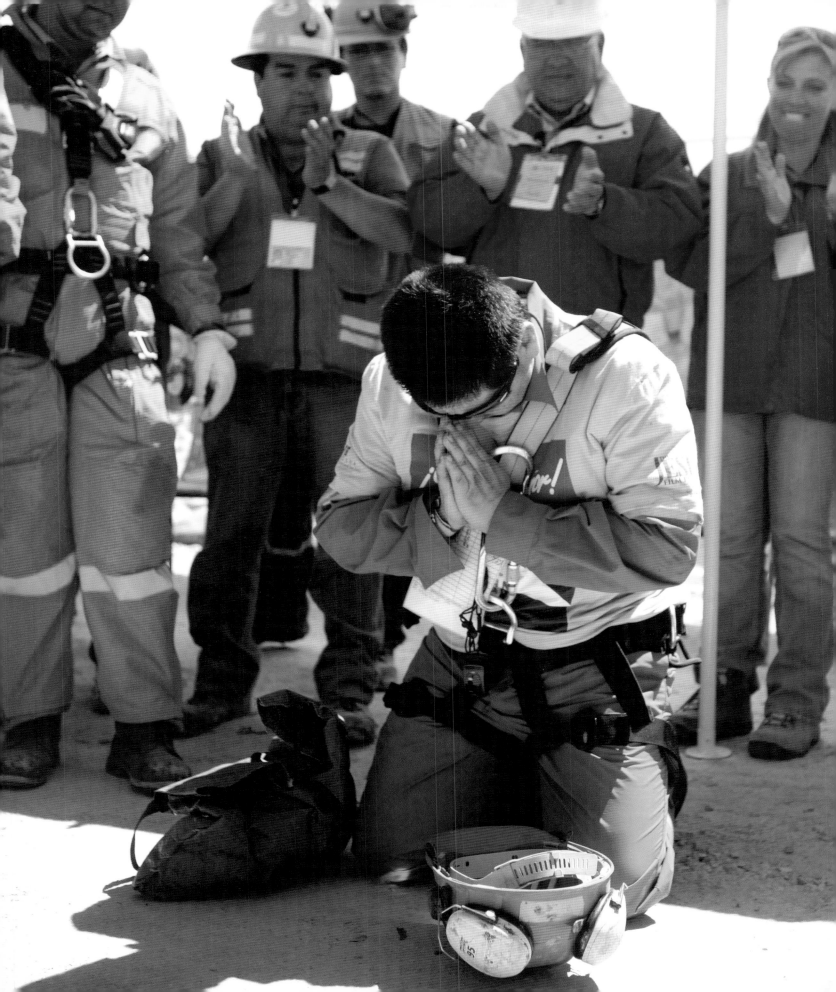

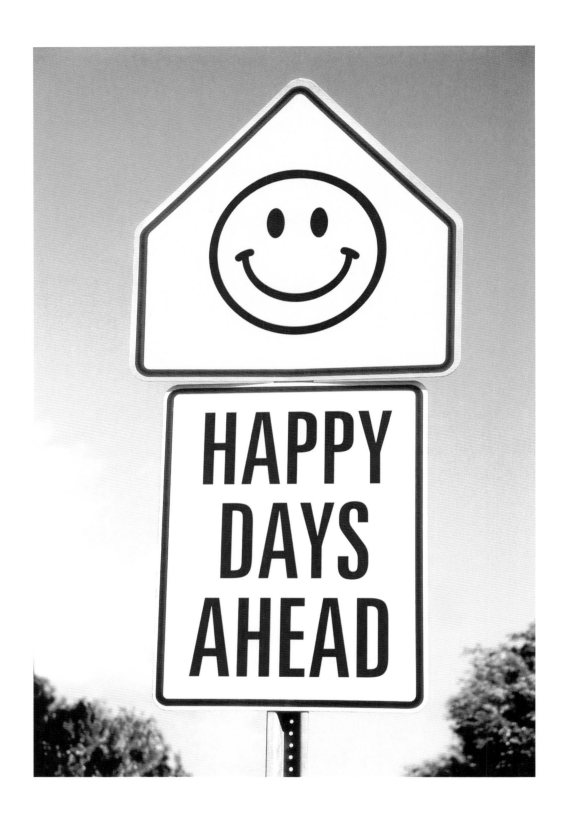

alive, 69 days after being trapped. The date—October 13, 2010.

THE IMPETUS TO KEEP GOING

What kept the men going? Social support, leadership, collaboration, discipline, a sense of humor—all these played vital roles. Most important, however, were optimism and hope.

Those working above ground were based in Camp Hope. Those in the bowels of the earth emphasized hope, faith, and optimism in their communication with rescuers and families. The pope and other religious leaders prayed for them. One of the miners had the amazing experience of watching his wife give birth to their daughter through a visual communication setup during the rescue operation. The parents called her Hope, because they, along with the other miners and their families, never lost hope. The youngest miner, Jimmy Sanchez, shared his hopes and thoughts in a letter: "I want to eat so many things. I'm hungrier than ever. All these days I've been dreaming about my mom cooking for me. That will happen soon. After the bad comes the good."[1]

It was a frightening and harrowing experience for all concerned, but running throughout their amazing story are the threads of optimism and hope—indispensable ingredients of a full, healthy, and happy life.

Optimism and hope make all the difference.

DEFINING OPTIMISM

What is optimism? There are many synonyms and related words: "happiness," "hope," "joyfulness," "positive attitude," "high spirits," and "cheerfulness," among others. Optimism has been defined as an enduring tendency to expect good personal outcomes in the future.[2] This fits with the Oxford dictionary definition, which describes optimism as an inclination to "hopefulness and confidence."[3] Hope and optimism will therefore be used interchangeably in this chapter.

Two people looking out the same window may see different things. The optimist, for example, may see beautiful stars that brighten the night; the pessimist may see dirty mud, which further depresses the mood. Through the eyes of an optimist the glass is seen as half full; through the eyes of the pessimist the glass is seen as half empty. Optimism is the face of our faith, and it is built on hope and trust in God, and belief that He can work things out for our best. This is based on the verses: "We know that in all things God works for the good of those who love him" (Rom. 8:28, NIV) and "God is faithful; he will not let you be tempted beyond what you can bear. But when you are tempted, he will also provide a way out so that you can endure it" (1 Cor. 10:13, NIV).

The optimist may have peace and even joy when things do not turn out the way he or she had wanted. In this life we experience brokenness, sickness, and even death; yet through all this, we may know an equanimity and peace that are beyond human understanding or expectation. By exercising the choice to be optimistic, we can enjoy wholeness even in our human brokenness. (And we all are broken in some way or another, be it physically, mentally, emotionally, or spiritually.)

HOPE WITHOUT HEALING

She was in her late 30s and a mother of three. Her diagnosis was that of melanoma (malignancy of the skin), which had now spread throughout her body despite treatment to keep the tumor under control. She had been through much in her quest for a cure, including participation in two clinical trials. The tumor had shown a mild response to one of the treatments, but at the cost of many hospitalizations, severe fatigue, a punctured lung, and severe infections. When the cancer again was found to be out of control, she eagerly enrolled in a third clinical study. This was to be different from the previous experiences—this was an early phase trial, and any benefits would be for the research. She was unlikely to benefit herself. This particular study required major surgery prior to taking the experimental medication.

The evening before the operation when asked if she had additional questions, she smiled and stated that

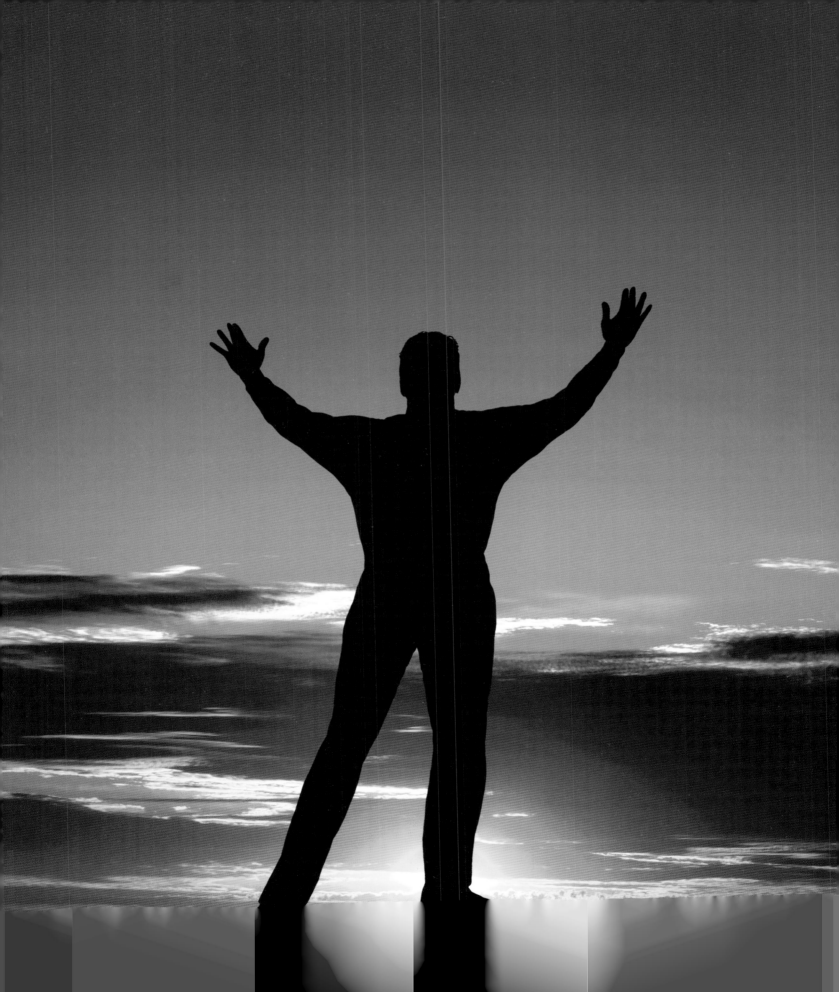

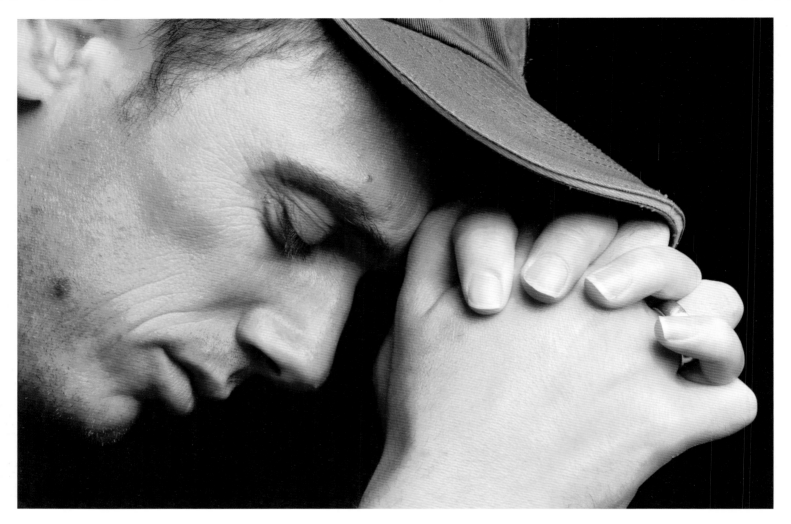

Optimism is the face of our faith, and it is built on hope and trust in God, and belief that He can work things out for our best.

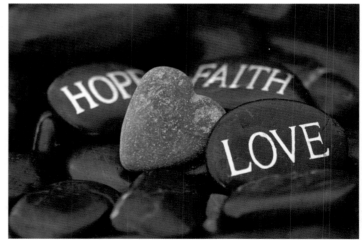

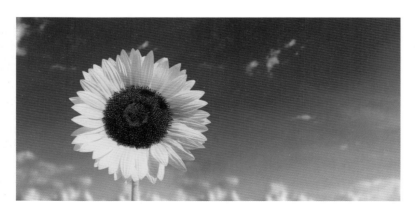

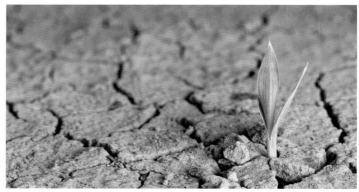

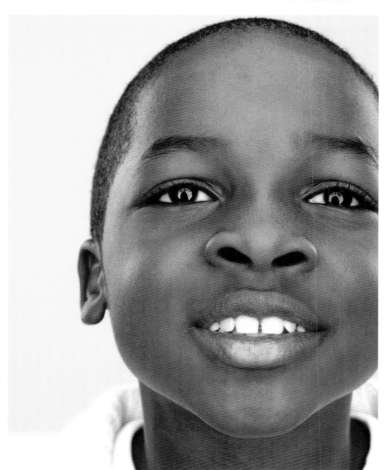
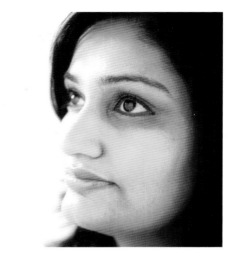
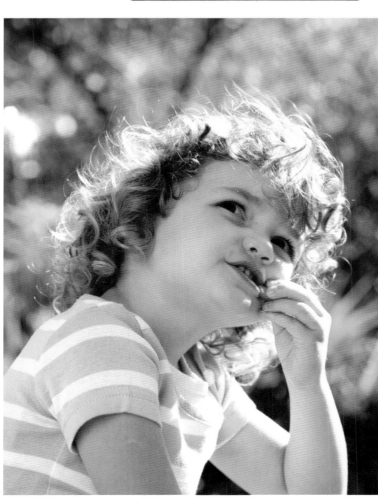
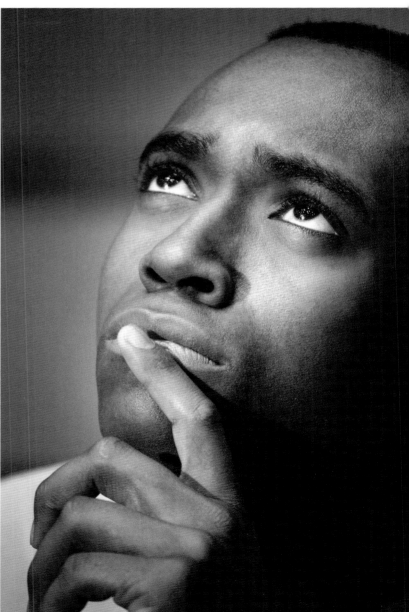

she didn't and that having been through this before she knew what she was letting herself in for. Then in a lowered tone she added that she was a mother and would do anything to be able to have even just a little more time with her children. The attending staff members were in awe of her selfless courage. They were also impressed that her optimism, although based on false hopes in a hopeless situation, had to be of some benefit to a person in her position. She died one year later—the tumor did not respond to the experimental treatment.

This sad but also inspirational experience confirms what we know so well—things don't always turn out the way we would like them to. Many of us need help making the choice to be optimistic, particularly under difficult circumstances. Family and other social support is both helpful and essential in this process. Pessimists tend to believe that bad events will last a long time, and they often relinquish the idea that situations will improve. The approach of the optimist, on the other hand, is to view a negative event as a temporary setback and be spurred on to try harder. Sometimes the realistic approach, which takes challenges and problems into account, may be viewed as pessimism; at the same time, a realistic optimist nurtures hope and perseverance, choosing to believe and work toward the improvement of circumstances and situations. "A pessi-mist sees the difficulty in every opportunity," Sir Winston Churchill said. "An optimist sees the opportunity in every difficulty."

A substantial amount of research demonstrates that hope and optimism are associated with better mental and physical health. Additionally, people with higher levels of optimism have more effective coping mechanisms.[4] In 2007 *New Scientist* published a fascinating article describing the demonstration of an area deep in the middle of the brain that is thought to be important in signaling and generating cheerful thoughts. Dr. Phelps and colleagues conducted these groundbreaking studies using magnetic resonance imaging (MRI), which may help us to better understand states of cheerfulness and depression even on an anatomical basis.[5]

LAUGHTER IS GOOD MEDICINE

In the late 1970s Norman Cousins authored a book entitled *Anatomy of an Illness*.[6] In it he describes his own experience with a debilitating illness and how, when medications failed to alleviate his pain and discomfort, he decided to watch humorous movies that elicited spontaneous and genuine laughter. To his delight and surprise he enjoyed physical and emotional improvement and ultimately returned to normal functioning.

Since that time much research has focused on the positive effects of

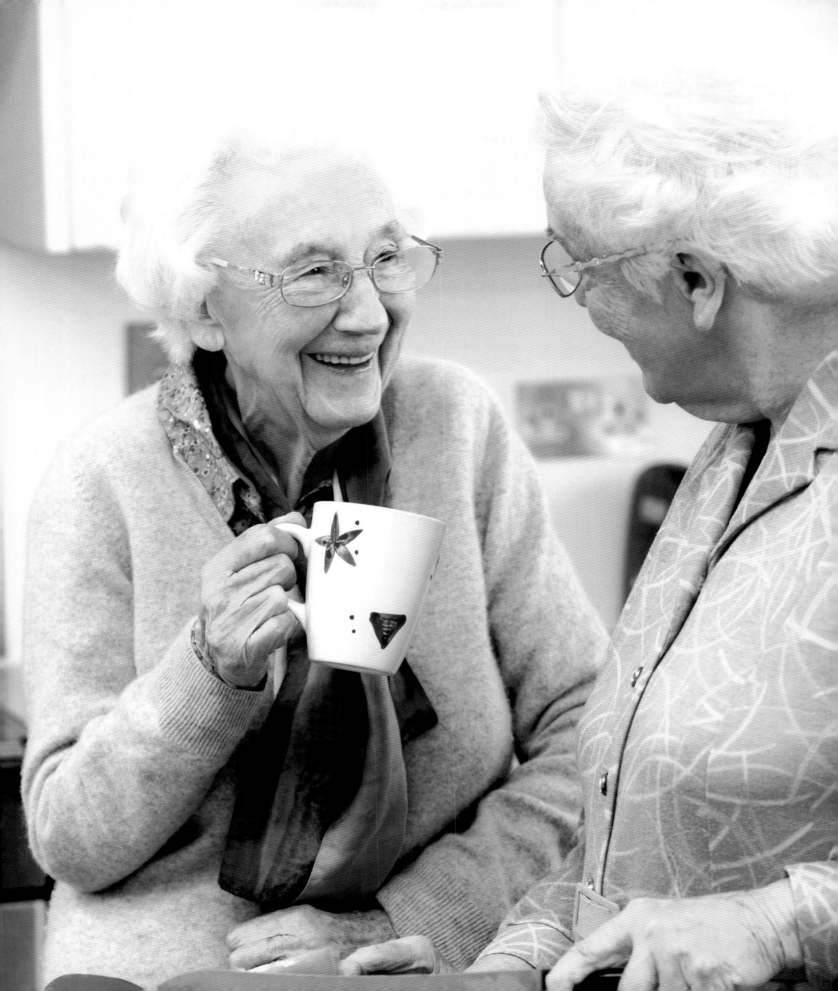

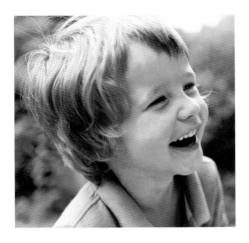 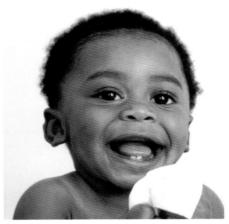 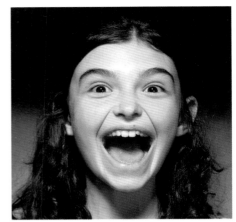

genuine, relaxing laughter showing significant benefits to health, including an increased pain tolerance.[7] Laughter triggers an uptake of endorphins, one of the brain chemicals responsible for the feeling of well-being as well as reducing pain.

We are fearfully and wonderfully made! No wonder the Bible says: "A cheerful heart is good medicine, but a crushed spirit dries the bones" (Prov. 17:22, NIV).

So what may hearty laughter do for our bodies? It can:

- exercise the lungs.
- stimulate the circulatory system.
- increase the oxygen intake into the lungs, which is then distributed by the blood to the cells.
- act as an internal jogger: The heart rate, breathing, and circulation will speed up after good and hearty laughter.

Subsequently, the pulse rate and blood pressure will decrease, and the skeletal muscles may then become relaxed.

Studies show that each time a person is happy and has laughed genuinely (not forced, superficial laughter), the sympathetic nervous system is stimulated, which in turn produces catecholamines. These catecholamines then stimulate the anterior lobe of the pituitary gland to produce endorphins, which:

- are the body's natural opiates that soothe and relax the mind. They can relieve pain more effectively than morphine.
- elevate the mood.
- may increase the activity of the immune cells.

Laughter is surely a powerful medicine.

The twentieth-century lifestyle studies by Drs. Belloc and Breslow from the Department of Public Health, Berkeley, California, reinforce that longevity has a close connection with the happy disposition of people. This study involved 6,928 adult residents of Alameda County, and the results showed that those who were generally unhappy had a death rate 57 percent higher than those who were generally very happy.[8] It's not always possible to be happy and laughing, but a positive

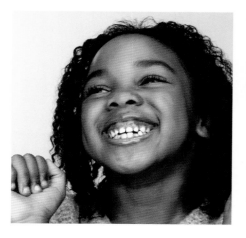 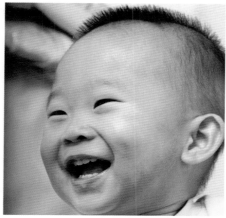 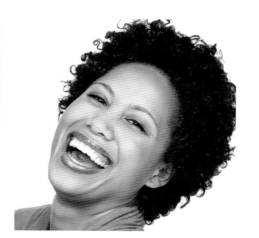

attitude can be cultivated—and studies show that a positive, optimistic attitude carries beneficial effects.

We can be happy and experience genuine laughter, especially when we completely trust God, knowing that He is in control of our lives no matter what the circumstances may be.

POSITIVE THOUGHTS

Another interesting study was conducted by Dr. David McClelland, who showed a group of students a photograph of a couple sitting on a bench by a river. He requested that each student write a story about this couple to gain greater insight into each student's subconscious perceptions and projections. He found that those who wrote stories depicting the positive outlook they had of this couple, envisioning them as enjoying a happy, trusting relationship, helping each other, respecting each other, and sharing warm, loving feelings with each other, demonstrated higher levels of immune antibodies and also reported fewer infectious diseases during the preceding year. Those who wrote stories depicting a negative outlook of the couple, in which they were seen to be manipulating, deceiving, or abandoning each other, demonstrated lower levels of immune antibodies and reported experiencing significantly more illness during the previous year. [9]

Nurturing positive thoughts and emotions about people and situations impacts our own personal well-being. It's also essential to note that our lives are not lived in a vacuum—we are social creatures. Social support and connectedness also strongly influence our emotional, spiritual, mental, and physical health. [10]

SUMMING UP OPTIMISM

The positive effects of hope and optimism impact human life at all ages and in many settings. Optimism significantly influences mental and physical well-being by helping to promote a healthful lifestyle as well as coping and adaptive responses/behaviors with more robust

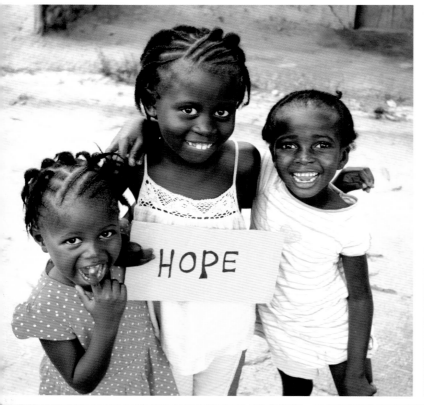

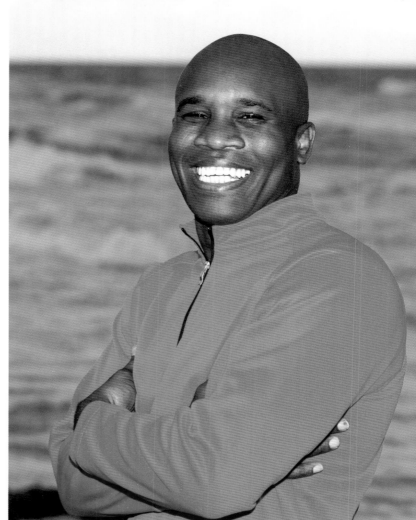

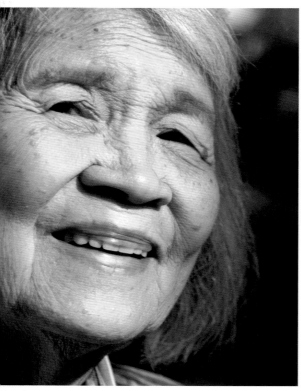

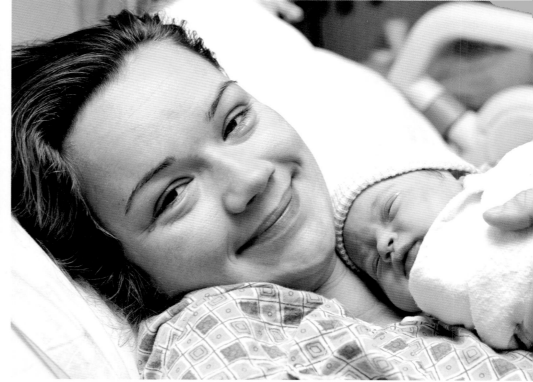

coping and problem-solving skills. These benefits also help to prevent burnout in such demanding situations as chronic-disease caregiving. Looking after Alzheimer's patients is one example of this.[11]

There will be times when we may feel just like the Chilean miners after the rockfall—trapped, buried alive by the events and circumstances that befall us. But we are never alone. We may choose to be optimistic, especially as we recall the wonderful promises of Scripture such as Lamentations 3:21-23: "Yet this I call to mind and therefore I have hope: Because of the Lord's great love we are not consumed, for His compassions never fail. They are new every morning; great is Your faithfulness" (NIV).

With such assurance we may celebrate life and enjoy wholeness, even in our present brokenness. Optimism and hope are truly the joy in life!

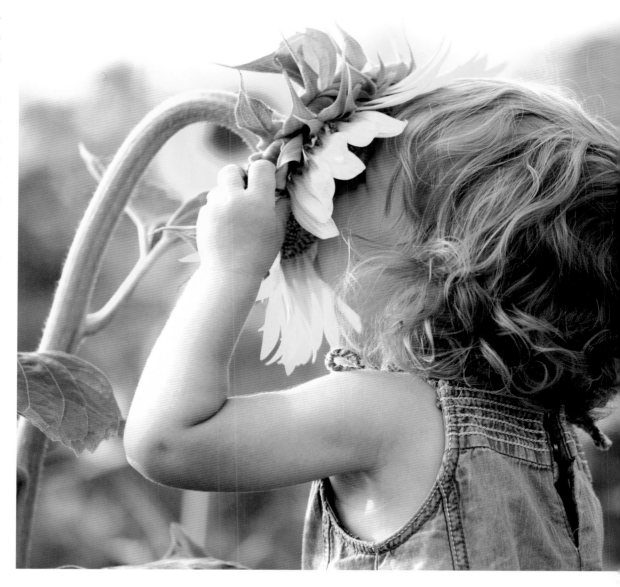

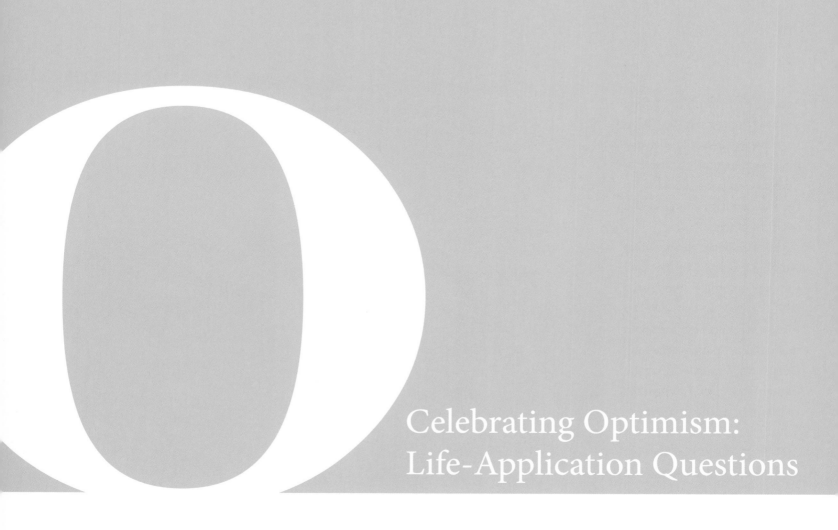

Celebrating Optimism: Life-Application Questions

Take the time to consider these questions and apply what you are learning to your life.

1 What devastating event have I experienced in my life that made me feel as if my world had caved in around me? Did I choose to have hope in that situation? What, if anything, gave me that hope and assurance? If something like that happens again, what extra sources of hope can I tap into? Which promises of Scripture will I choose to memorize?

2 In most situations am I more likely to see the positive aspects or the negative ones? How can I change my perspective to become more optimistic, even while being realistic? What can I do so that I look for opportunities rather than difficulties?

3 When was the last time I experienced genuine, relaxing laughter, so that my lungs got exercise and my whole body did a little internal jogging? What triggered this event? What choices will put me in this situation more often? How do I make wise decisions in the choice of my friends, what I view on TV, what I read? How can I adjust my view of God, so that I can be joyful without feeling guilty?

GROUP DISCUSSION

4 Stories abound of missionaries who faced incredible odds. Their children died of malaria; they lived in very poor housing; they had to travel under difficult circumstances. Some were often ridiculed; others saw very few results of their labors. Many were single with very few chances to meet with friends. And all this while living thousands of miles from their homeland and families. In spite of the hardships and sacrifices, however, they did it joyfully and willingly. What gave them that optimism? What choices can we make in order to be selfless and optimistic like that?

5 How can we nurture positive thoughts and emotions about people and situations? How can we balance the bad news we hear with the good news of the gospel? Do the stories we read or the movies we watch give us confidence that God is in control and working toward the salvation of the world and a better world to come?

How can I change my perspective to become more optimistic, even while being realistic?

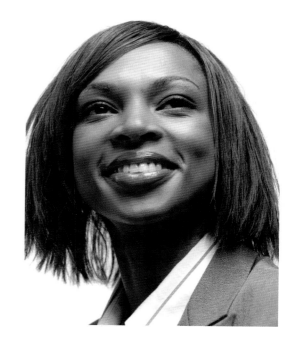

Celebrating Nutrition

Imagine with me that you have just come into possession of the sports car of your dreams! Money was no object in its design and manufacture. Even the smallest detail had been tended to with meticulous care. On the outside, the doors and fenders are aligned perfectly. The finish sparkles with perfection. You pop the hood and are greeted with the sight of an engine that is made with the craftsmanship of a fine Swiss watch. When you open the car door you savor the smell of soft, subtle leather. As you sink into the wonderfully padded seats and turn the ignition key to start the engine, you hear the purr from the powerful engine. The moment has come for you to take this—your car—for a drive!

After a few hours of pure enjoyment you notice that the fuel gauge is showing close to empty, so you pull into the first gas station you find. Looking in the owner's manual you see that the manufacturer has recommended only premium fuel for the high-compression engine. You decide, however, that any grade fuel will do and fill it with "regular" instead. After all, you think, they look and smell the same. Later, when you check the engine oil, you top it up with a little water.

With that kind of care, how long do you think your dream car will last?

Our bodies are far more beautiful and complex than the finest machine ever made by humans. Like a fine

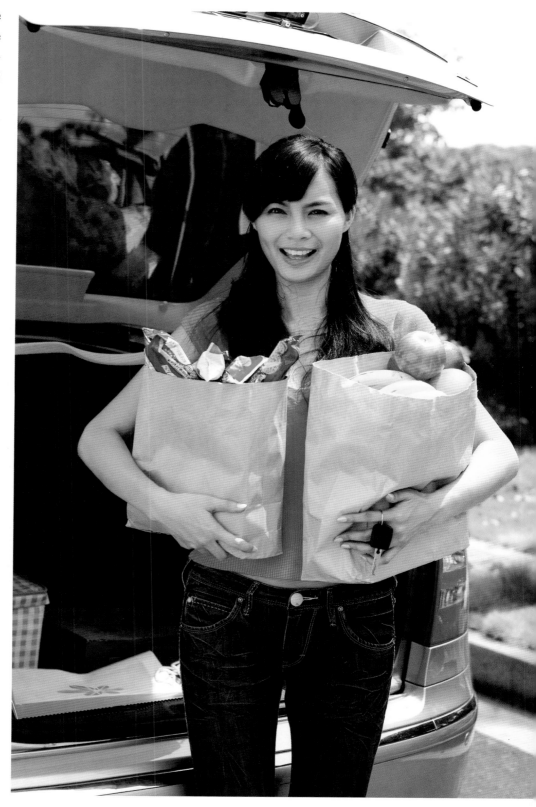

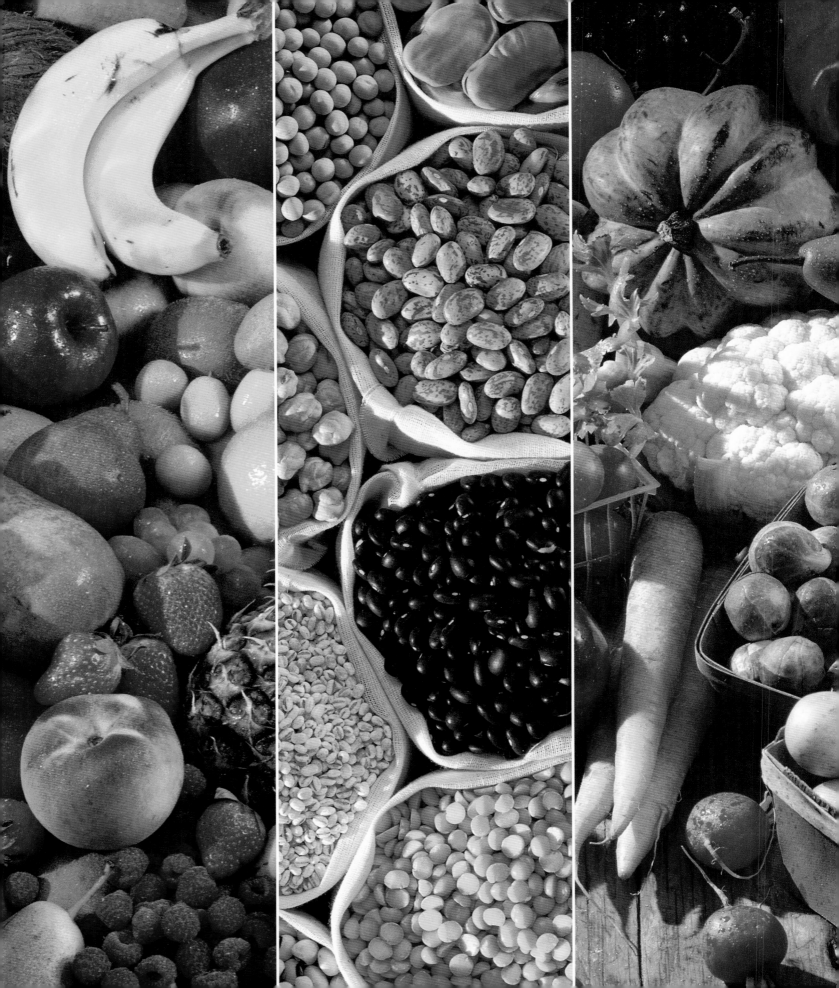

sports car, our bodies need fuel to power our lives, and that fuel comes from the food we eat. A balanced diet chosen from the best foods will provide the essential nutrients needed for growth, maintenance, and energy. If we choose low-quality foods or do not eat enough of even the best foods, the body machinery will suffer. Too much food may result in obesity, and excessive amounts of some nutrients may cause toxicity.

THE RIGHT BODY FUEL

Why wait for a special occasion to celebrate? Shouldn't we celebrate every meal with healthful food choices? In each meal one can enjoy the cornucopia of nutrient-dense, whole-grain breads and cereals, along with rich, colorful fruits and vegetables containing abundant amounts of vitamins, minerals, dietary fibers, and phytochemicals. Enjoy essential fats in crunchy nuts and seeds, bone-building calcium from low-fat milk or a fortified soymilk, and healthful proteins from satisfying legumes (beans, peas, and lentils) seasoned delicately with herbs and small amounts of salt, sugar, and vegetable oil as needed. These energizing, body-building foods consumed daily in appropriate quantities can reduce the risk of cancer, coronary heart disease, hypertension, intestinal disease, obesity, and osteoporosis. We can truly celebrate at every meal because of the abundance of good food God has given us!

UNDERSTANDING NUTRITION

Many people think that choosing good nutrition is difficult, and understanding it even harder. Both tasks, however, are really very simple. Let's start with the "understanding" part.

Our bodies get the nutrients we need from the food we eat as the food is digested and assimilated in a fantastic process that begins in the mouth, moves to the stomach, then to the small intestines, and finally to the large bowel. The nutrients our bodies need include:

Carbohydrates: The largest portion of our diet should come from these in as unrefined a form as possible. Whole grains, legumes, fruits, and vegetables are rich in these. There are approximately 4 kcal (a unit used to express the amount of energy contained in food) per gram in carbohydrates.

Proteins: Every cell in the body contains proteins. Tissue repair and growth require them. While almost all foods contain some protein, particularly good sources are milk, eggs, and other animal products. Legumes are excellent plant sources. Each gram of protein yields 4 kcal.

Fats: These are a concentrated source of energy. We often get too much fat in our diet because we like the flavor it imparts to foods (e.g., boiled or baked potatoes versus French fries).

Vitamins (fat soluble and water soluble), minerals, and trace minerals: These are essential for growth and health.

Antioxidants and phytochemicals: These substances protect the body from disease and some of the effects of aging. They are found primarily in whole grains, fruits, vegetables, and nuts.

ESSENTIAL FOOD GROUPS

There are five essential food groups. When we eat foods wisely chosen in appropriate amounts from all five groups, we will meet our optimal nutrient needs. Here are the five groups:

CEREALS AND GRAINS: These should form the foundation of our diet. They include whole-grain breads, pastas, rice, and corn. They are rich in dietary fiber and complex carbohydrates, as well as an array of vitamins and minerals when taken from unrefined (not white) sources. Depending on a person's age, weight, and activity levels, 6 to 12 servings from this group should be consumed each day.

FRUITS AND VEGETABLES: These foods come in a wide variety of colors, flavors, and textures and are the richest sources of protective phytochemicals, antioxidants, and many vitamins and minerals. Depending on body size, age, and activity levels, at least 5 to 10 servings of these foods chosen from a range of colors should be consumed daily. Many people seem to prefer fruits over vegetables, but we need a balance of both. Foods in this group that are the deepest in color often have the largest amounts of phytochemicals and antioxidants. Fruit juices should be limited to no more than 1 small serving per day.

LEGUMES, NUTS, AND SEEDS: Legumes such as beans, peas, and lentils are an important source of good protein, along with minerals, vitamins, and other protective elements. Three to 5 servings of these should be included in the daily diet, depending on a person's age and weight. Nuts and seeds are excellent sources of essential fats, but because they are a concentrated source of calories, they should be limited to no more than 1 to 2 servings per day. Nonvegetarians would include fish, fowl, and meat in this group, but should consume only moderate amounts.

DAIRY AND EGGS (OR FORTIFIED EQUIVALENTS): These animal sources of food provide many important nutrients, including calcium and vitamin B_{12}. Vitamin B_{12} is found only in animal products and prevents pernicious anemia and neurological disorders. It also promotes normal cellular division. Individuals who choose not to consume any animal products need to eat sufficient foods fortified with vitamin B_{12} or take it in supplement form. It's very important to read the food labels of the equivalent foods to make certain that they are adequately fortified. Deficiency symptoms of vitamin B_{12} can take 4 to 6 years to develop after all intake has been stopped. By the time problems have been discovered, permanent damage may already have occurred.

FATS, OILS, SWEETS, AND SALT: These foods are required only in small amounts. The essential fats and sodium are necessary for optimum health. Iodine is a necessary trace mineral and is easily supplied if iodized salt is used; it also can be obtained from sea salt, seaweed, or a supplement. Refined sugar is not required for good health, but small amounts add palatability and flavor to our foods.

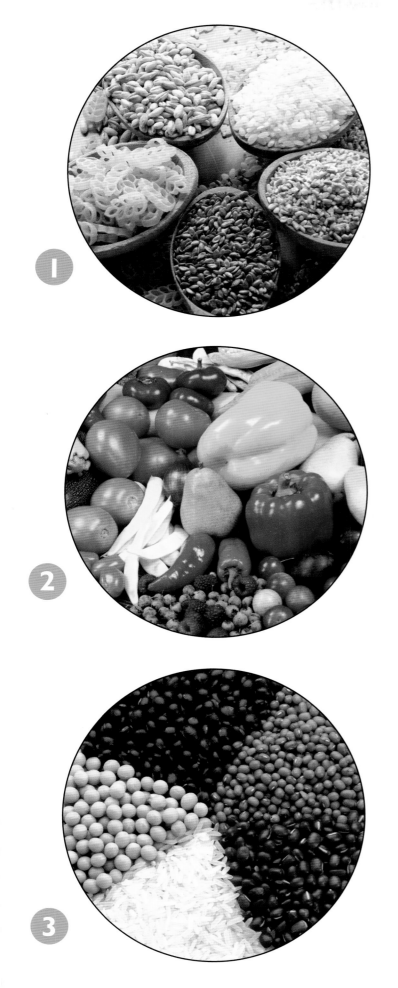

1

2

3

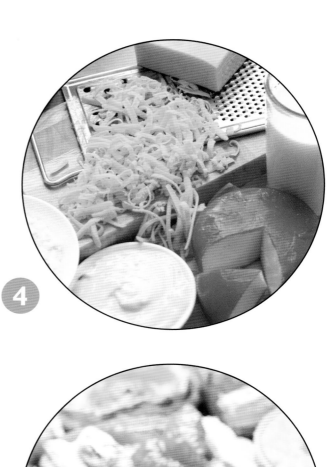

4

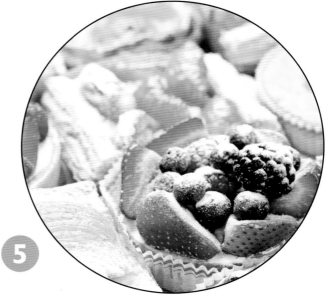

5

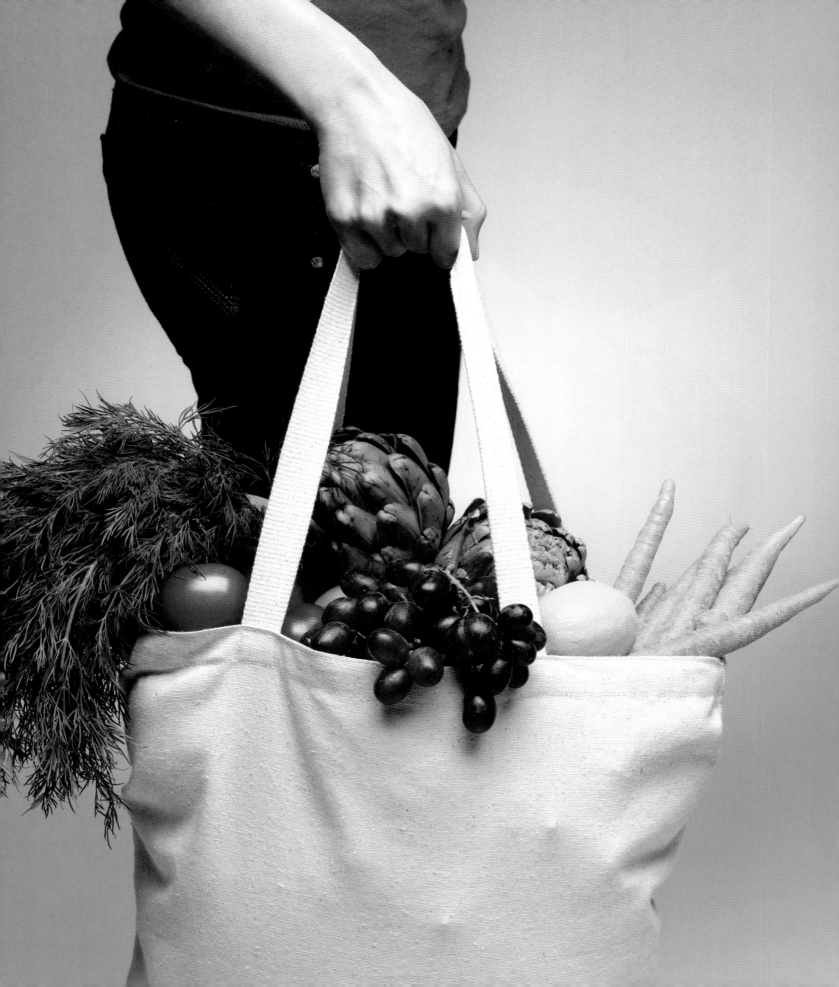

One of the most important keys to eating a balanced plant-based diet is selecting a variety of foods whose color, texture, and flavor add interest to the diet. These foods are best when consumed as they come from nature: not refined, not pulled apart, not fractionated. Whole foods should be the goal.

"Use plant foods as the foundation of your meals. . . . Eating a variety of grains (especially whole-grains), fruits and vegetables is the basis of healthful eating."[1] This recommendation has been simplified in the 2010 "Dietary Guidelines for Americans" to "Make half your plate fruits and vegetables."[2]

Today the world is recognizing the advantages of a vegetarian diet:

▪ Low in fat, particularly saturated fat

▪ No cholesterol (with a total vegetarian diet)

▪ High in dietary fiber

▪ Low in refined sugar (need to avoid highly sweetened items, even if from plant foods)

▪ Contains rich sources of vitamins and minerals

▪ Contains high amounts of protective substances such as phytochemicals, antioxidants, etc.

GUIDING PRINCIPLES OF FOOD CHOICES

A healthful diet needs to be based on sound principles that guide the food choices we make. We would like to suggest five:

1 VARIETY: Perhaps the most important principle of eating right is selecting a variety of foods from the five groups discussed earlier in this chapter (cereals and grains; fruits and vegetables; legumes, nuts, and seeds; dairy and eggs or equivalents; and fats, oils, and salt). This ensures a wide range of nutrients to support a healthy body, and the various textures, tastes, and colors enhance the pleasure of eating.

2 QUALITY: Choose the majority of your food from whole foods—not refined foods. These foods are nutrient-dense rather than calorie-dense.

3 BALANCE: Obesity is a growing problem worldwide. There needs to be a balance between the amount of energy we eat (foods) and the energy we expend (physical activity) if we are to maintain a healthy weight.

4 MODERATION: Some important components of a healthful diet need to be eaten only in small amounts. These would include fats and salt. We require adequate amounts of the essential fats. Fats are also the vehicle for fat-soluble vitamins. We also need small amounts of salt to maintain our electrolytes.

5 AVOIDANCE: Highly refined foods that often have large amounts of their nutritional elements removed should be avoided, as should foods and beverages that have no nutritional value (alcohol, coffee, and sodas).

Many excellent online tools are available that allow you to track and analyze what you eat every day. One of the best is SuperTracker,[3] which is free for anyone to use.

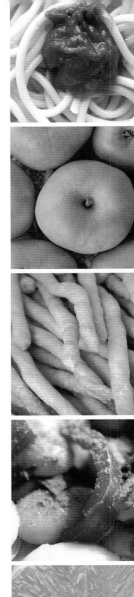
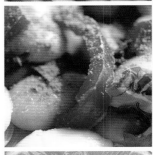
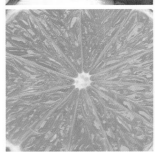
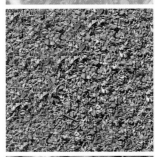
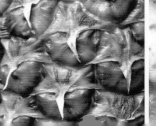

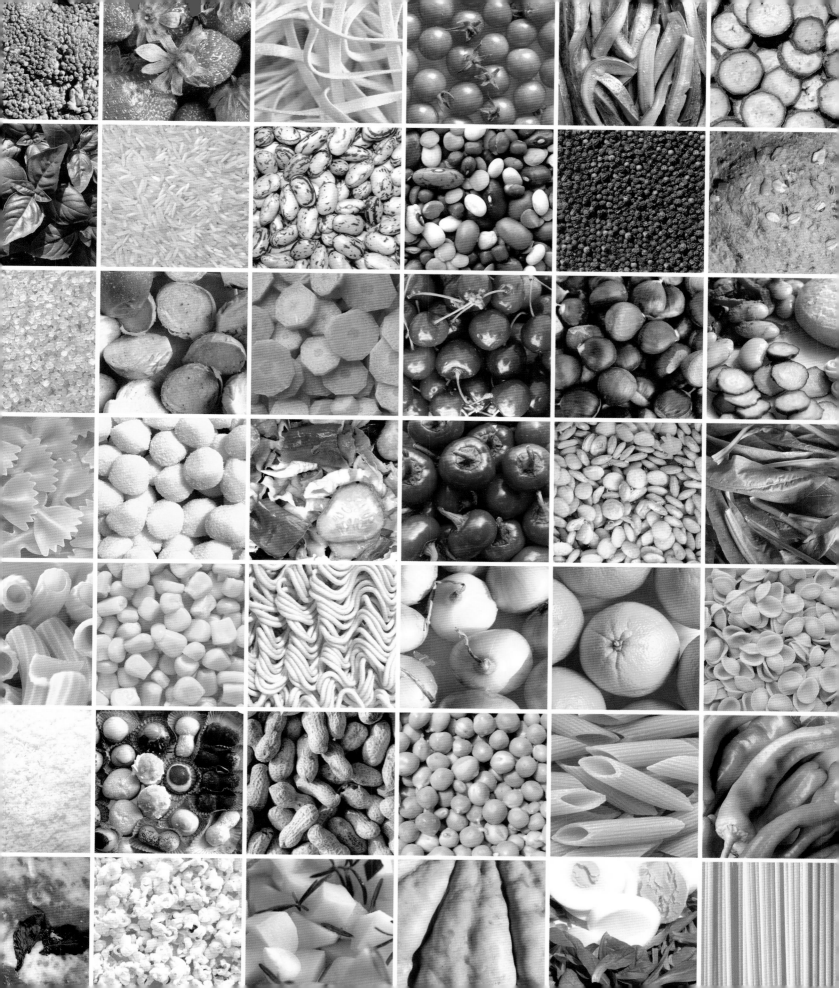

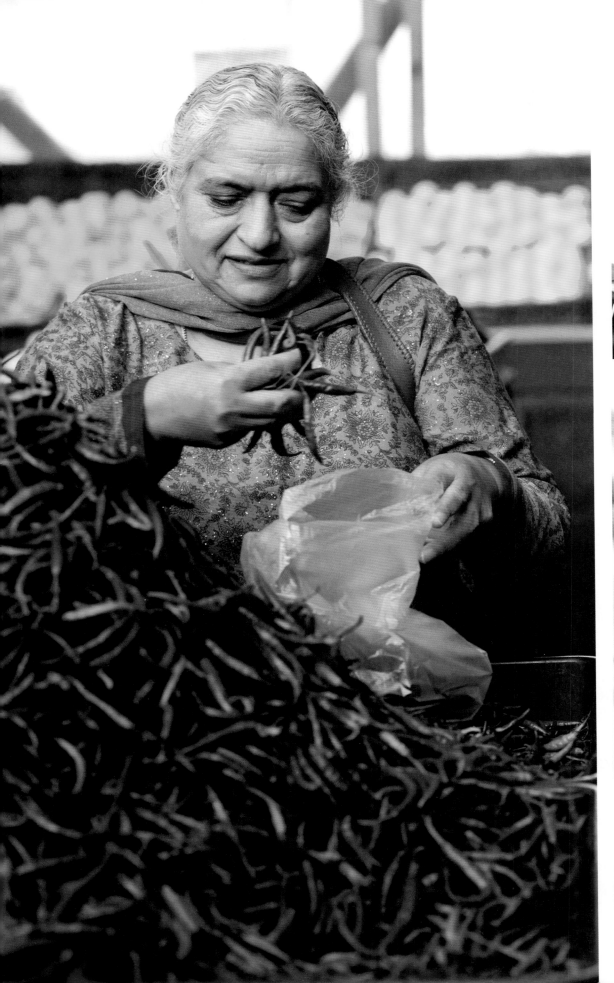
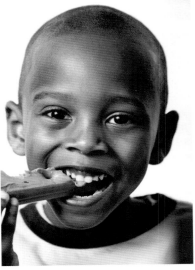
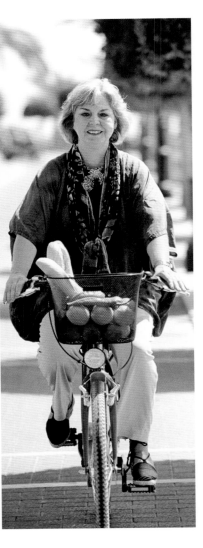

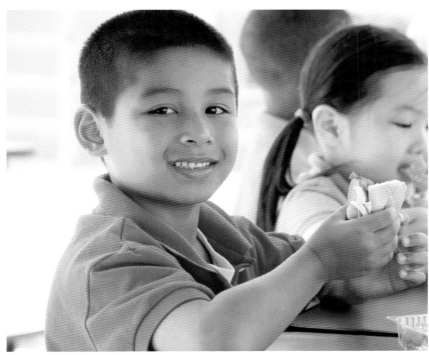

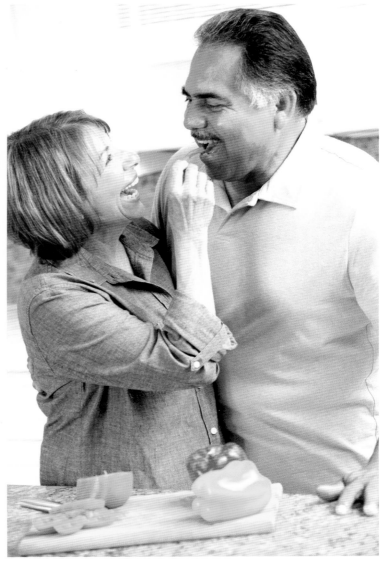

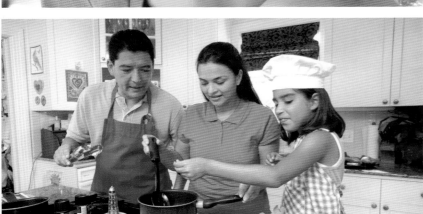

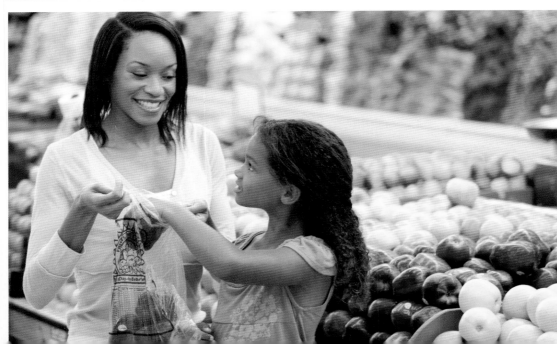

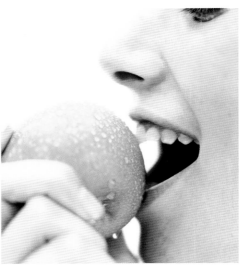

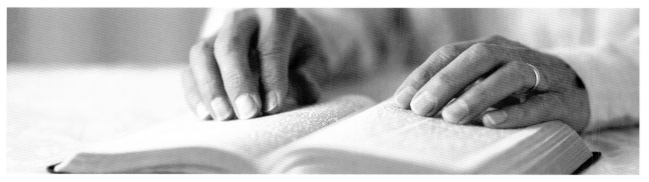

SPIRITUAL FOOD

A healthful diet can increase lifespan and the quality of life. God loves us and desires that we lead healthy, productive, and happy lives. We can celebrate His goodness as we appropriately enjoy the many products of the earth that He has given us.

Just as we require physical food each day, we also need to feed the inner person on spiritual food. We should not neglect to make a daily practice of feeding on God's Word. We have emphasized the need for variety, balance, and flavor in the foods we consume, but we require balance in our spiritual food, as well. We can feast on God's Word by contemplating His wonderful promises, reading inspirational stories and exhortations, and spending time daily in prayer. These practices will help us to grow spiritually as well as physically. Balance and control in life come from the steady application of the lessons learned in the reading of His Word.

Let us do these things with praise in our hearts for the energy and health that God provides.

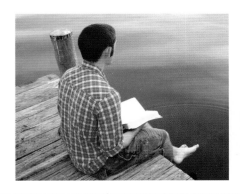
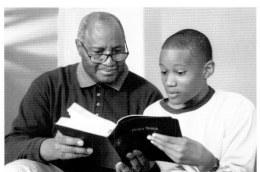
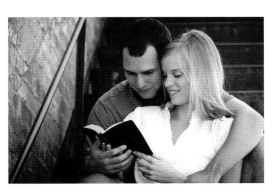

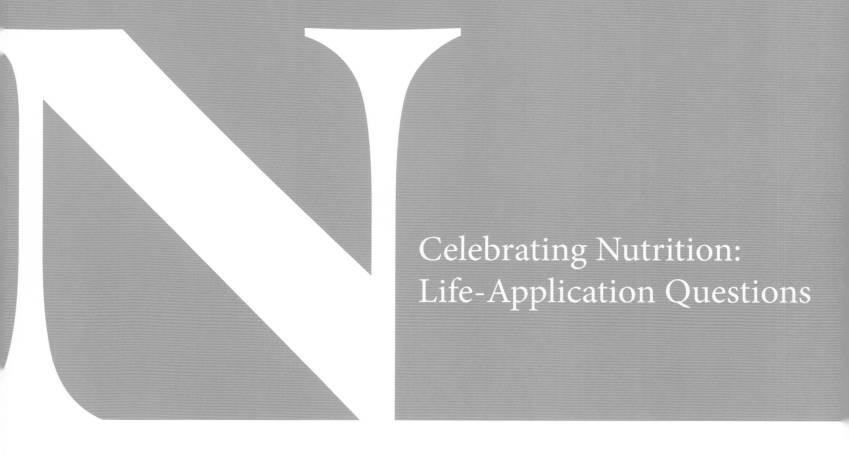

Celebrating Nutrition: Life-Application Questions

Take the time to consider these questions and apply what you are learning to your life.

1 What foods did I choose for my three most recent meals? What proportion of what I ate consisted of cereals and grains; fruits and vegetables; legumes, nuts, and seeds; dairy and eggs? Did I make wise choices, or did I take too much of one group and too little of another? How much of my plate contained fruits and vegetables? How colorful was my plate? Did I have enough of the richly colored vegetables?

2 What portion of these meals consisted of highly processed products? Which of these can I start cutting back on, and which of the cereals, grains, and legumes can I enjoy eating more regularly?

3 How much did I consume of the essential fats and oils? Did I eat enough to ensure that I got the fat-soluble vitamins I need? Do I use too much fat or oil with my meals? How can I still have palatable food without using so much fat? How can I use herbs more creatively? Should I try to use more fresh foods?

4 Do I routinely use too much salt? Do I reach for the saltshaker without having first tasted my food? Have I read the labels of the processed foods I use to ensure that they are not hiding a great deal of salt (sodium) that would be harmful?

5 Is my body getting adequate amounts of vitamin B_{12}? How do I make sure I supplement these before I develop symptoms of irreversible neurological damage? Do I get adequate calcium in my diet, or am I at risk of bone loss?

6 How do I balance my intake of energy in the food I eat with my output of energy in physical activity? Do I weigh myself regularly to ensure that I am maintaining a healthful weight? Do I need to lose some excess weight? What "tricks" can aid me in my choices? How does using a smaller plate help me to lose weight? Do I need to choose more fiber-rich foods?

GROUP DISCUSSION

7 Susie's friend Nathan noticed that Susie was a vegetarian. He asked her about the advantages of such a lifestyle. What reasons could Susie give for her choice, and what should she emphasize the most? If a nonvegetarian invites a vegetarian to his home for a meal but expresses concern about how he could cook a meal without meat, what simple, balanced recipes would be easy for him to prepare? What about inviting him to church-run cooking schools?

8 Do we place too much emphasis on our own dietary habits? Do we want healthy bodies so we can glorify God? Do we praise Him with the spiritual diets that we choose?

Do I need to choose more fiber-rich foods?

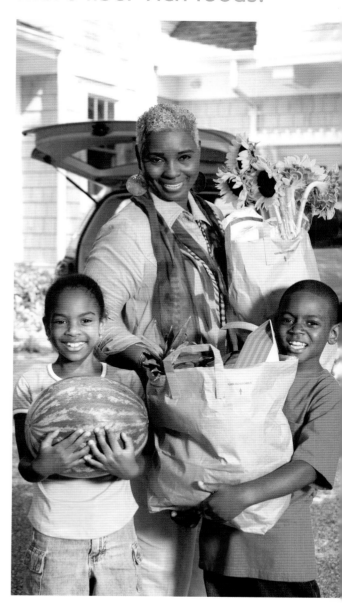

Celebrating
Social Support

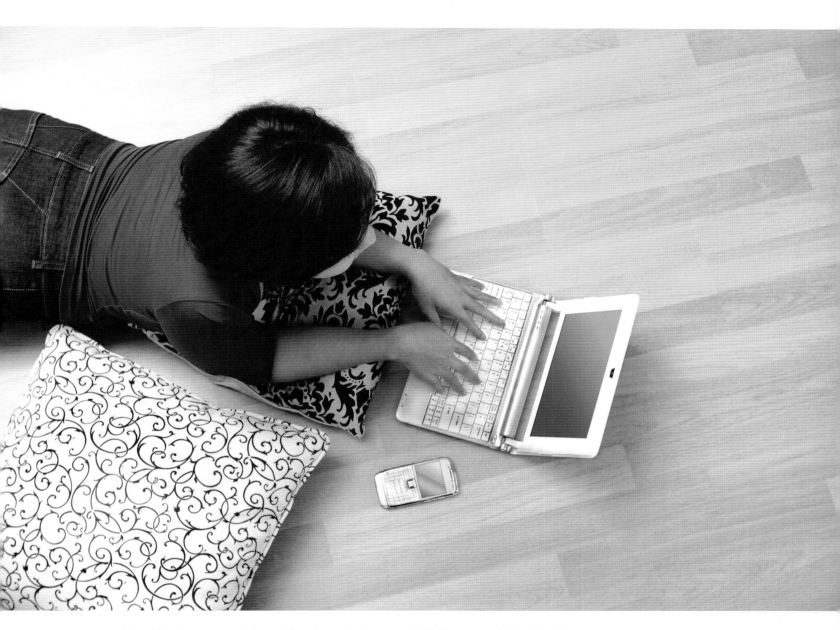

Julia Neuberger, a rabbi of South London Liberal Synagogue and one of the first two female rabbis in the United Kingdom, was also chair of the Commission on the Future of Volunteering (2006-2008) and the prime minister's Champion for Volunteering (2007-2009). Communicating well with others is a vital part of her work and ministry. In the January 1, 2010, issue of *The Guardian*, however, she wrote, "One change I'd like to see in the coming year is a move away from social networking sites. The rise of MySpace, Facebook, LinkedIn et al. has been an important cultural shift of the last decade, with many of us now using the web to make 'friends' and meet possible partners. There is nothing wrong with that in

Love is as essential to the growth of a human being as is food.

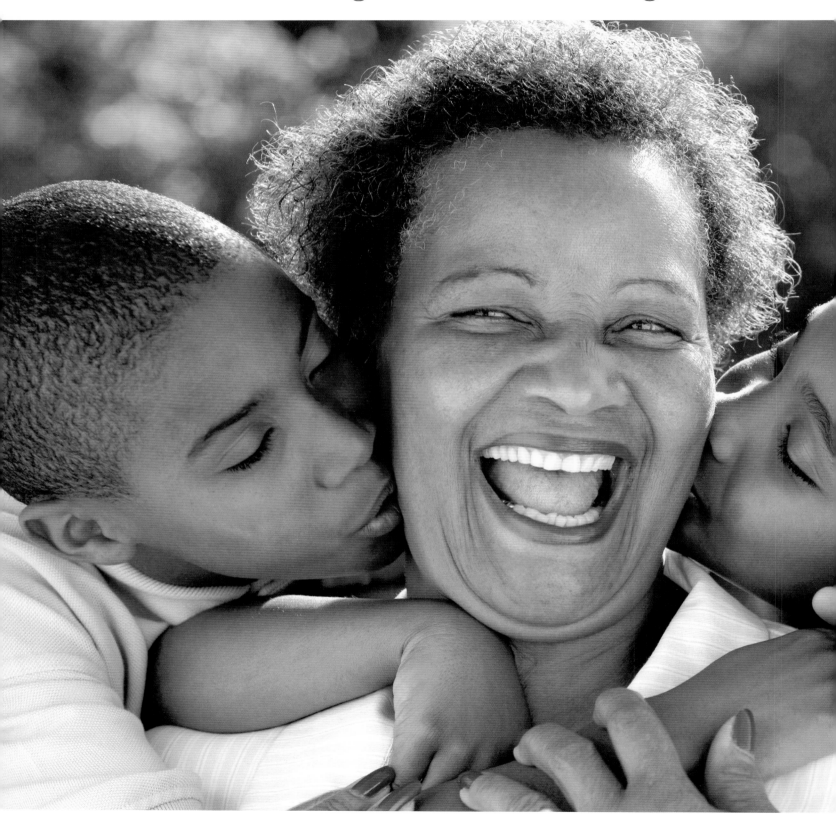

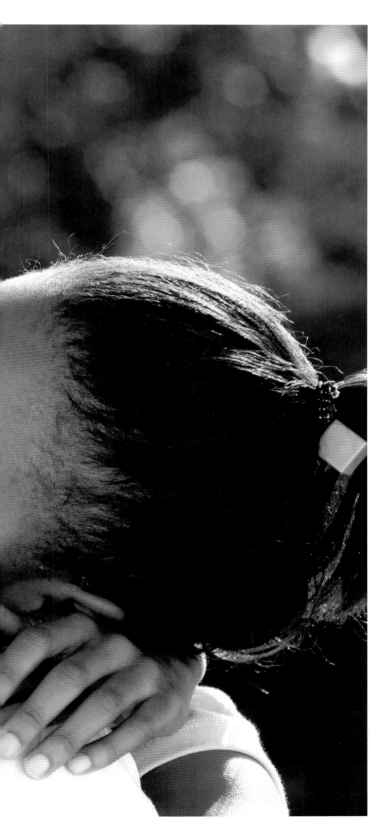

principle, provided they realize that the internet, however much it has transformed our lives for the better, is no substitute for meeting people, getting out there and making friends. . . . Those sites can only make initial connections; they cannot begin to develop the depth of real friendships, of real connectedness."[1]

Social support is a vital factor in the health of individuals and society. Selfishness and pride have separated nations, kingdoms, tribes, communities, and families. Selfish interests drive wedges between us. True religion teaches that all nations are one in the eyes of God and that there is unity in the family of humankind. Regardless of our diversity, we are all one by creation, and we should respect the dignity of others in all societies. Such unity encourages a willingness to provide service to one another.

Why are support and willingness to provide service to others so vital to our daily living? As psychologist Abraham Maslow observed, love is as essential to the growth of a human being as is food.[2]

According to psychologists Sheldon Cohen and S. Leonard Syme,[3] social support has direct and indirect effects. Direct effects benefit both the giver and the recipient of social support and can be measured by comparing groups that receive and do not receive such support.

Supporting one another helps us cope with stress. It's important to realize that we can be our own worst enemies by refusing the support of others. Our attitudes may influence how we respond to the efforts of others to support us.

Psychologists L. F. Berkman and T. Glass stated that social support affects a person's health through pathways such as mental outlook, health habits, and the way the body works:[4]

◼ Our friends may have a positive or negative influence on us. Supportive friends build self-esteem and self-efficacy. Some friends subtly undermine and depreciate us.

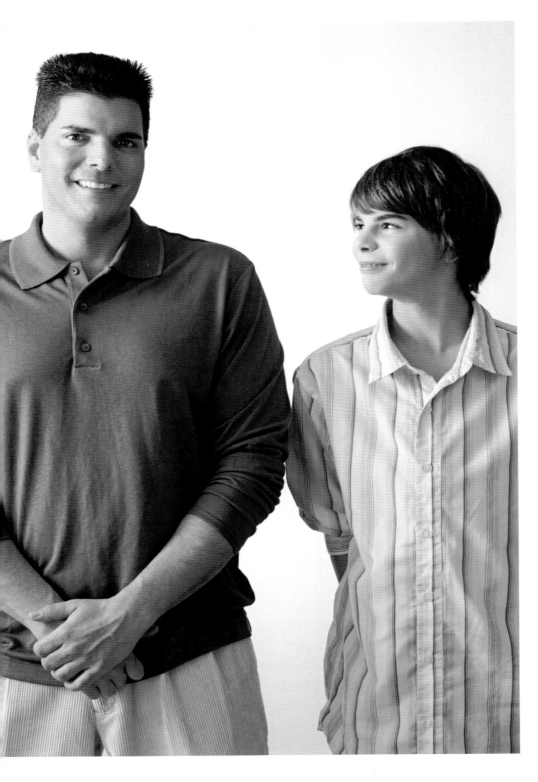

Friends who themselves have unhealthful habits or even a lack of friends may lead us to seek comfort in unhealthful activities such as smoking, drinking, and overeating.

Support from friends strengthens our coping abilities and reduces our stress. Criticism and negative attitudes affect our health possibly through the effect on the immune or cardiovascular system.

SUPPORT OF FAMILY AND FRIENDS

According to E. Stice, J. Ragan, and P. Randall, family support is the most important factor in the lives of adolescents. Many have experienced the support of family and friends as a commitment on their part to love, nurture, and help them. Adolescents have high expectations of parents, and inadequate parental support increases the risk of adolescent depression. They become disappointed and confused when the anticipated help and positive reinforcement from parents are missing. The support of friends is also very important for adolescents.[5]

SUPPORT IN THE SCHOOL

School occupies a considerable amount of time in a youngster's life, so it's not surprising that the experience of young people in school will play an enormous role in their development. Such influence is probably second only to that of the home.

Psychologists V. Battistich and A. Horn studied an ethnically and socioeconomically diverse sample of 1,434 fifth- and sixth-grade students from 24 elementary schools throughout the United States.[6] They found that students in supportive settings enjoyed school more, were more academically motivated, and were far less involved in disruptive and delinquent behaviors and drug use. If students sensed "community"—opportunities to engage with others in school and other social groups, and participate in community activities—they flourished. It's important that our youth do more than merely survive adolescence, but blossom into wholesome adults.

SUPPORT IN THE FAITH-BASED COMMUNITY

The Commission on Children at Risk, a group of 33 children's doctors, research scientists, and mental health and youth service professionals, found considerable support for the role played by authoritative communities in health. These are communities that have a firm basis for belief in their sacred scriptures and from which they derive a value base. For adults, religious faith and

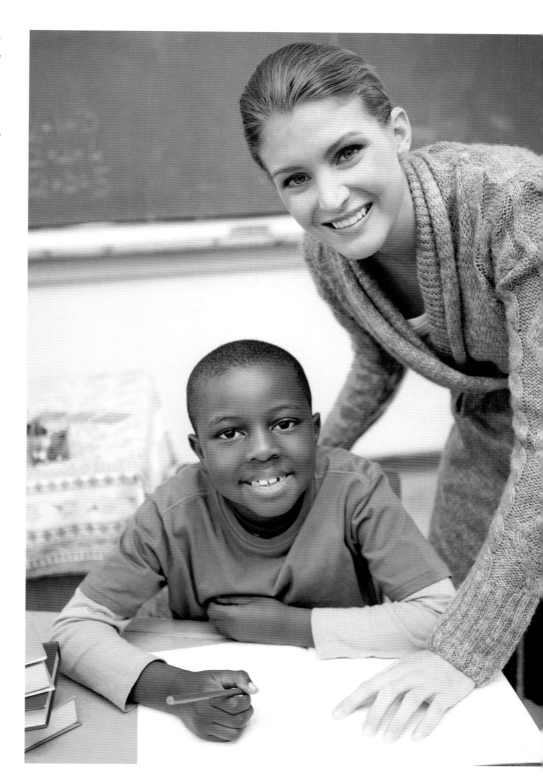

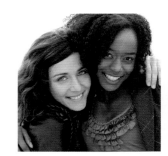
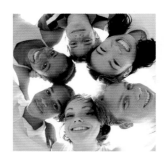
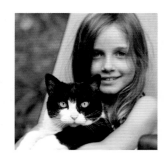
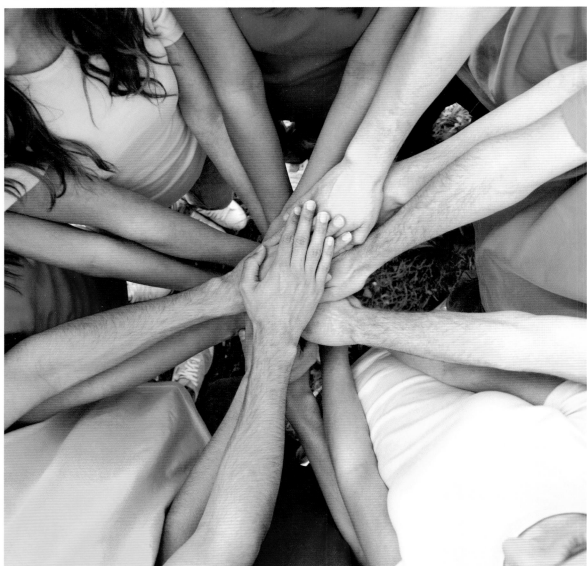
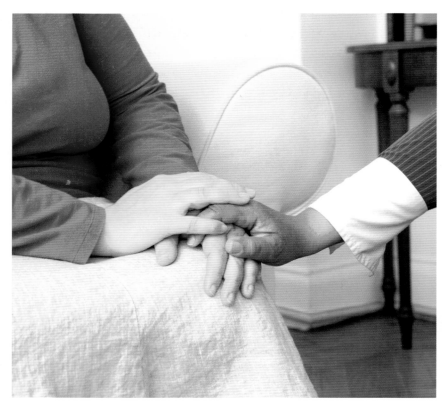
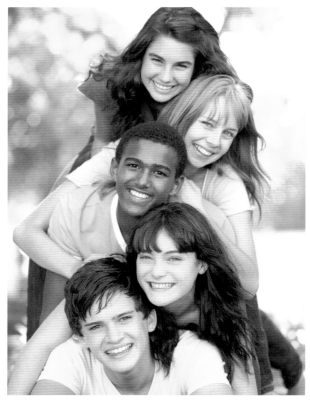

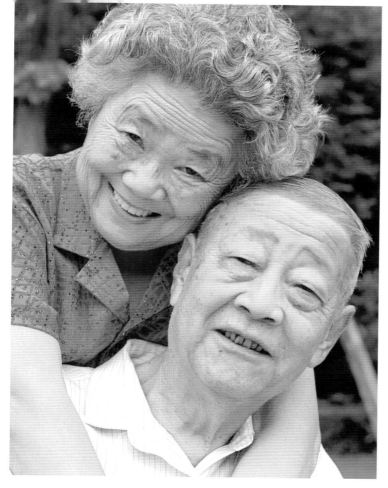

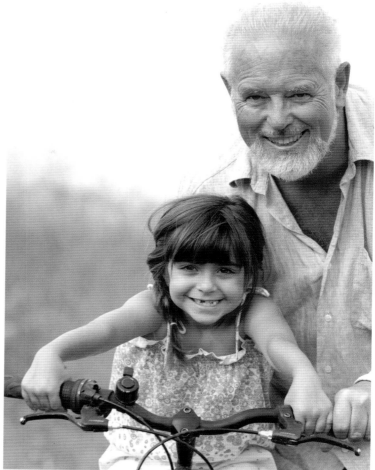

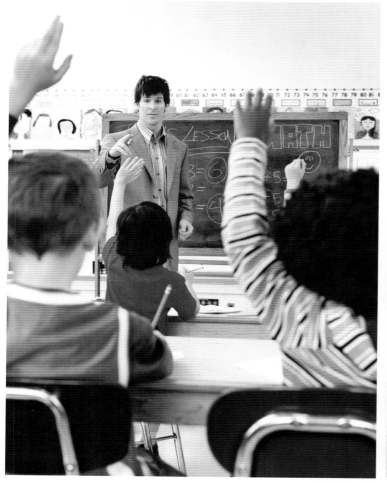

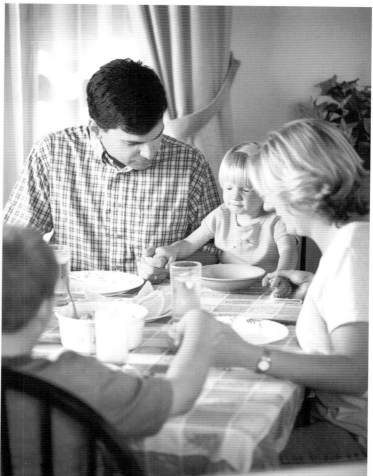

practice appear to have a sizable and consistent relationship with improved health and longevity, including less hypertension and depression, a lower risk of suicide, less criminal activity, and less use and abuse of drugs and alcohol.[7]

SOCIAL SUPPORT AND THE RECOVERY OF DISEASE

A study that is part of an eight-year investigative partnership between Vanderbilt University Medical Center and the Shanghai Institute of Preventive Medicine, beginning in 2002, was published in the *Journal of Clinical Oncology*. Meira Epplein et al. found that among 2,230 breast cancer survivors, women who scored highest on the social well-being quality-of-life scale had a 48-percent reduction in their risk of dying from cancer or having a cancer recurrence. Specifically, women reporting the highest satisfaction with marriage and family had a 43-percent risk reduction, and those with favorable interpersonal relationships had a 35-percent risk reduction.[8]

Social well-being in the first year after cancer diagnosis is an important prognostic factor for breast cancer recurrence or death, and some health professionals support the concept of designing breast cancer treatment to maintain or enhance social support soon after diagnosis is made in order to improve the outcome of the disease.[9]

There is plenty of research to convince us that surrounding ourselves with people who genuinely care about us can have a positive effect on our mental well-being. A strong social support network can be critical in helping us through the stress of tough times, whether we've had a bad day at work or a year filled with loss or chronic illness. Supportive family, friends, and coworkers are a very important part of our lives.

CARDIAC ARRHYTHMIA SUPPRESSION TRIAL

Social support definitely benefits the receiver, but what about the giver? More than 150 years ago Ellen G. White wrote that "doing good is a work that benefits both giver and receiver."[10] Science today agrees. Several studies by Drs. Siegel, Friedmann, Allen, and others, for example, printed in scientific journals, show that when a person provides love to their pets, they are healthier.

Back in the 1990s *The American Journal of Cardiology* published an interesting study conducted by Drs. Friedmann and Thomas known as the Cardiac Arrhythmia Suppression Trial (CAST).[11] The doctors studied men and women who had sustained a heart attack and had ir-

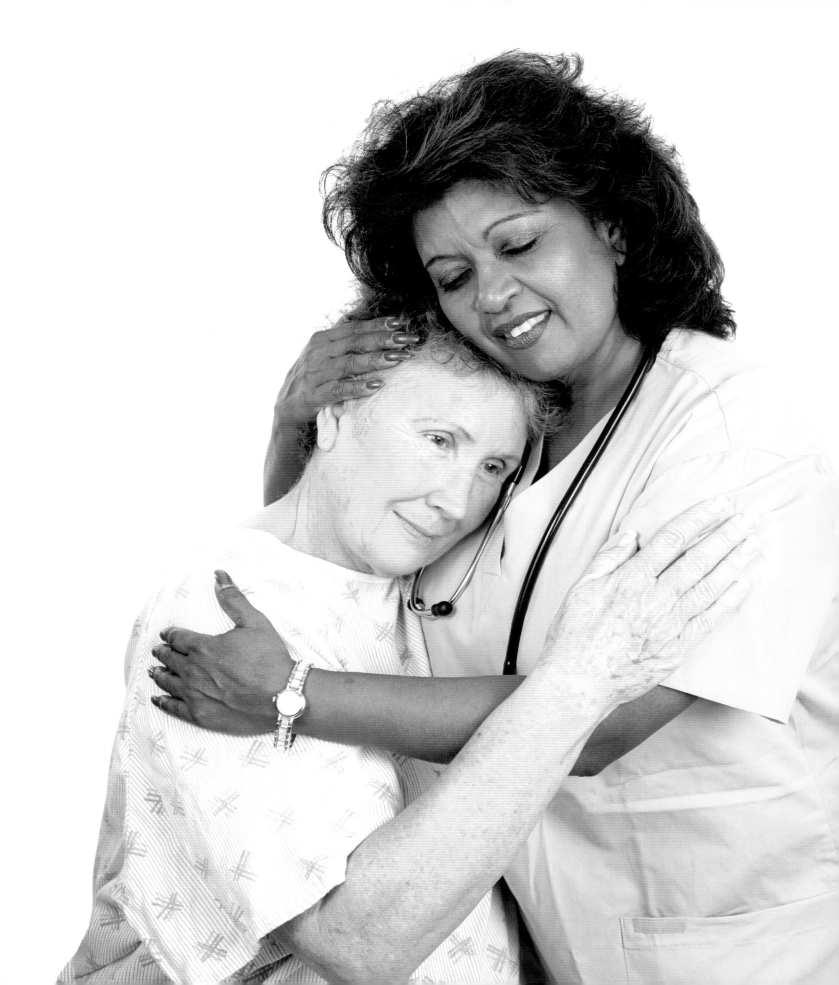

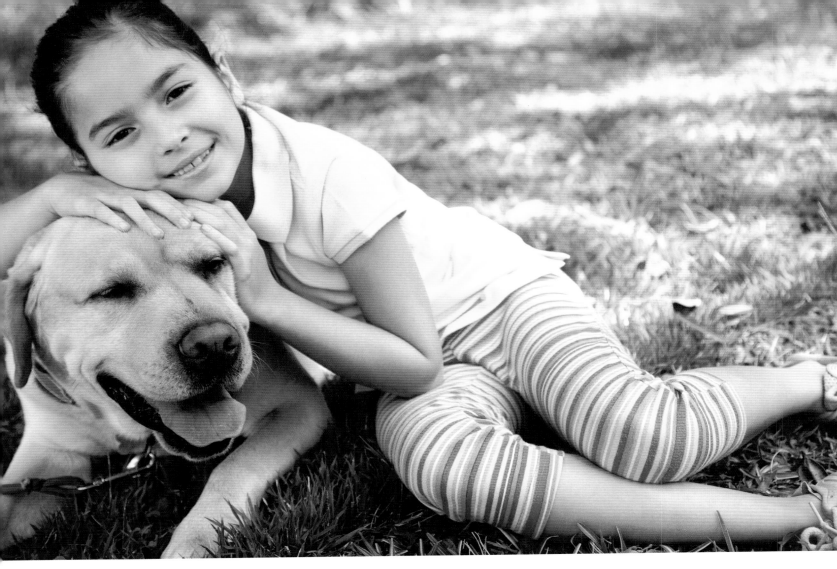

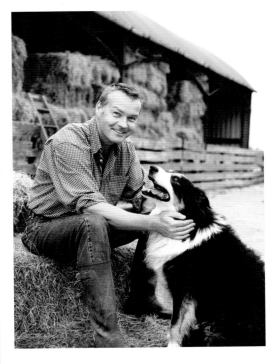

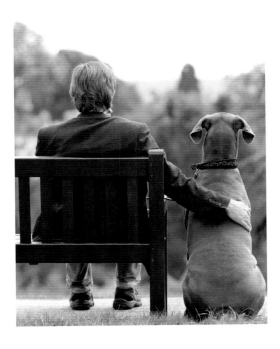

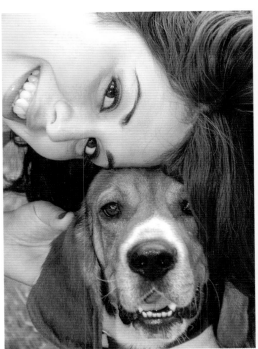

regular heartbeats. Here are surprising results from a substudy:

■ Only one of the 87 people (1.1 percent) who owned dogs died during the study.

■ Nineteen of the 282 people (6.7 percent) who did not own dogs died.

■ More than six times as many non-dog owners died compared to dog owners, which seems to indicate that dog owners benefit from providing loving support to their pets.

Ironically, the drugs tested in the main study—encainide and flecainide—actually caused an increase in cardiac deaths and had to be stopped prematurely. If these drugs had shown a sixfold decrease in deaths, you can be pretty sure that just about every doctor in the country would be prescribing them for patients with heart problems. When was the last time that your doctor gave you a prescription to improve your health by providing loving support to others or to a pet?

SOCIAL SUPPORT AT WORK

Ideally, social support should come from family, friends, and church members, but there also is a growing need for additional support from the workplace.

On average, adults spend one third of their day (a 24-hour period) sleeping and relaxing, one third with family and home responsibilities, and another one third with colleagues at work. With such a large time investment in work, individuals need social support in the workplace. As colleagues notice changes in personality and behavior or discover needs of coworkers—they may be struggling with family problems, school conflicts, or personal issues such addictions to harmful substances, gambling, or pornography—they can offer support. Friends at work sometimes can bridge the gap between employee and employer in tense situations or organize support teams. You can help to build a warm and caring climate by being genuinely interested in your coworkers' well-being.

Elizabeth Brondolo, Ph.D., a psychology professor at St. John's University in Stony Brook, New York, and her colleagues conducted an interesting study that discovered clear and measurable effects on blood pressure when people care for one another in the workplace. The study was conducted with 70 agents in New

York City who issue parking violations and traffic tickets. This can be a stressful job as motorists often insult, threaten, or curse agents. During the study the agents wore a small monitor that recorded heart rate and blood pressure throughout the day. They also kept a journal of their workday whereabouts and activities. At the day's end the agents completed a questionnaire that measured the emotional support they received from coworkers, immediate supervisors, and unit supervisors. "The more people felt supported by their co-workers, the smaller the increases in their blood pressure in the work environment." In fact, they had lower blood pressure during the most stressful times as well as throughout the workday.[12] This study definitely shows the importance of having social support at work.

Some of the most helpful support skills are very simple: listen to colleagues carefully and attentively, respect the other person's privacy and dignity, choose words wisely, be gentle and kind, keep a positive attitude, and avoid criticism. Treat the other person as you would want to be treated.[13]

WHAT IS A SOCIAL SUPPORT NETWORK?

A social support network comprises friends, family, and peers. It differs from other types of support groups in that it is not led by a mental health professional. Although both types of support groups can play important roles in times of stress, a social support network can be developed under conditions that are not stressful, thereby providing the comfort of knowing that our friends are there for us if we need them. Rather than formal meetings with an official leader, a social support group can simply be friends eating lunch together, neighbors chatting together, close relatives having a phone conversation, and even church fellowships. These all are ways to develop and foster lasting relationships with the people close to us.

Let's not wait for someone else to make the first move. If you meet a person who you think might become a good friend, invite that individual to join you for lunch or other casual activities. These activities can include volunteer groups in causes of mutual interest, or even exercising together at a gym or with a walking group.

THE IMPORTANCE OF GIVE AND TAKE

A successful relationship is a two-way street. The better a friend we are, the better our friends will be. Here are some suggestions for nurturing relationships:

■ **Stay in touch.** Answering phone calls, returning e-mails, and reciprocating invitations let people know we care.

■ **Don't compete.** Be happy instead of envious when friends succeed, and they'll celebrate our accomplishments in return.

■ **Be a good listener.** Find out what's important to your friends.

■ **Don't overdo it.** In our zeal to extend our social network, be careful not to

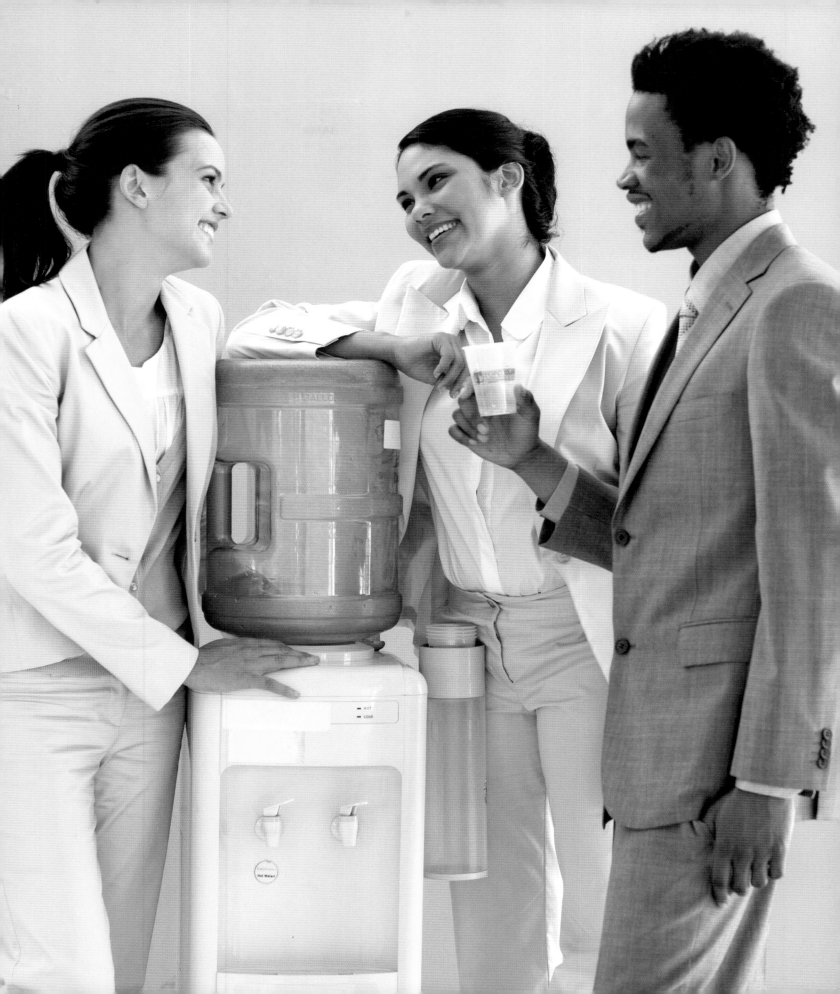

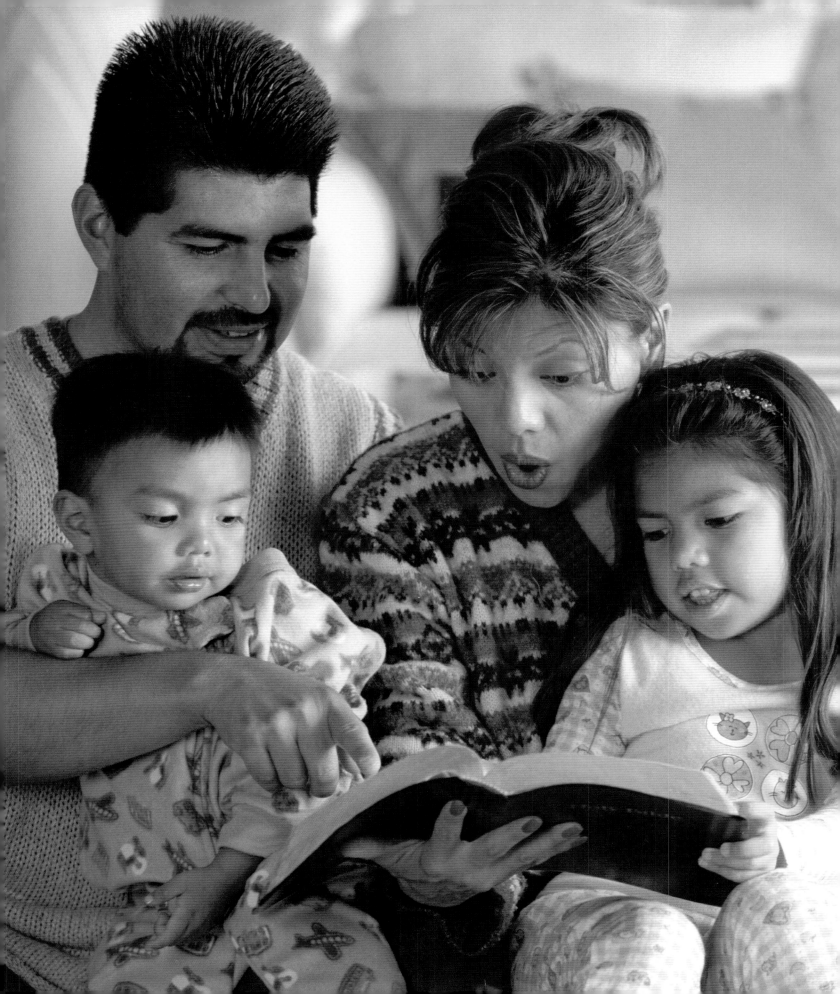

overwhelm friends and family with phone calls and e-mails.

■ **Appreciate friends and family.** Take time to say thank you and to express how important they are to us. Be there for them when they need support.

THE BOTTOM LINE

The purpose of building a social support network is to reduce stress levels, not add to them, so watch for situations that seem to drain our energy. For example, avoid spending too much time with someone who is constantly negative and critical. Similarly, steer clear of people involved in unhealthful behaviors such as alcohol or substance abuse, especially if you've struggled with these addictions yourself.

Taking the time to build a social support network is a wise investment not only in our mental well-being but also in our physical health and longevity. Those who enjoy high levels of social support stay healthier and live longer than those who don't. Let's start making more friends or improving the relationships we already have. Whether you are the one receiving the support or the one providing encouragement, you will reap a plethora of rewards.

A BIBLICAL APPROACH

In light of the benefits of social support, this statement makes much sense: "Christian kindness and earnest consecration are constantly to be manifest in the life."[14]

Having a meaningful relationship with the Lord will produce loving relationships with others and a desire to give them genuine support. We will appreciate one another as children of God, regardless of our backgrounds. We will not have to worry about what to say or do, because as we have a relationship with God, we truly will love one another, serve one another, strengthen and encourage one another, forgive one another, and pray for one another.

The social support we give and receive is very important to our overall health and well-being. Let us therefore live a life of praise to God by genuinely caring about the welfare of others and giving thanks for all things to Him who made us.

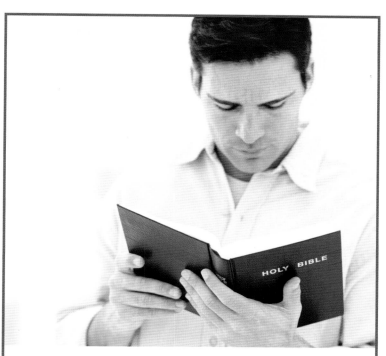

There are many Bible verses that provide specific instruction on how to practice kindness and to express loving social support to one another. Here are some examples:

New Testament
■ Love one another (John 13:35).
■ Forgive one another (Col. 3:13).
■ Accept/receive one another (Rom. 15:7).
■ Pray for one another (James 5:16).
■ Comfort one another (1 Thess. 4:18).
■ Fellowship with one another (1 John 1:7).
■ Be kind to one another (Eph. 4:32).
■ Show compassion to one another (1 Pet. 3:8).
■ Be hospitable to one another (1 Pet. 4:9).

Old Testament
■ Be hospitable to strangers (Gen. 18:2-5).
■ Do not pass along false reports (Exod. 23:1).
■ Do what is right (Mic. 6:8).
■ Honor your parents (Exod. 20:12).
■ Respect your neighbors (Exod. 20:13-17).
■ Love your neighbors (Lev. 19:18).
■ Real friends stick closer than a brother (Prov. 18:24).

Celebrating Social Support: Life-Application Questions

Take the time to consider these questions and apply what you are learning to your life.

1 Who are the members of my social support network from my family, school, work, church, and community? Thinking of each one of these people, whom should I look to and associate with most when I need encouragement and positive reinforcement? With whom should I spend less time because of the self-destructive behaviors they practice?

234

2 How can I develop deeper relationships with family and friends than is possible to attain through using the social networking sites on the Internet? How well do I listen to them? Do I remember the situations they are facing well enough to ask about how things are going? How often do I reach out to them compared to how often they contact me?

3 Who in my family, school, work, church, and community requires emotional support when they are coping with stressful situations? How do I coach them to see the opportunities rather than the difficulties? How can I develop confidence and hope in my Savior and His working out everything for the good and share that optimism and trust?

GROUP DISCUSSION

4 Harold has a coworker and good friend who does much the same work that he does. Recently his friend put forward an idea that earned the approval of top management and resulted in his being promoted. Some of his other colleagues are complaining that everyone in the department contributed to his success. How should his colleagues have reacted in such a situation? Why were they jealous of his success? In what ways can they rejoice with him?

5 When do we feel happiest: when we are with people who are supporting and serving us, or when we are serving others? How can we balance our need for support from others and the goal of service that contributes to the well-being of others and our own sense of being valued? What specific activities can we become involved in that will widen social support networks and provide opportunities of service?

When do I feel happiest: when I am with people who are supporting and serving me, or when I am serving others?

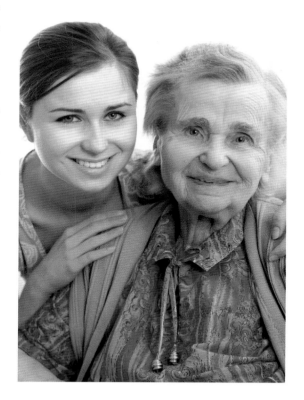

References

CHOICES

[1] Roland Huntford, *The Last Place on Earth—Scott and Amundsen's Race to the South Pole* (New York: Random House, Inc., 1999).

[2] N.B. Belloc, L. Breslow, "Relationship of physical health status and health practices," *Preventive Medicine,* August 1972, 1 (3):409-421.

[3] Ibid.

EXERCISE

[1] "An Exercise Story"; http://nihseniorhealth.gov/stories/ca_grace.html. Accessed online April 4, 2012.

[2] U.S. Department of Health and Human Services (2008), *2008 Physical Activity Guidelines for Americans,* pp. 9-12. For online version go to www.Health.gov/paguidelines.

[3] "Effect of Physical Activity and Diet on the Treatment of Metabolic Syndrome"; http://www.bioportfolio.com/resources/trial/75943/Effect-Of-Physical-Activity-And-Diet-On-The-Treatment-Of-Metabolic-Syndrome.html. Accessed April 20, 2012.

[4] "Your Guide to Physical Activity"; http://www.nhlbi.nih.gov/health/public/heart/obesity/phy_active.pdf. Accessed online April 4, 2012.

[5] D. O'Conner, M. Crowe, W. Spinks (2005), "Effects of static stretching on leg capacity during cycling," *Turin,* 46 (1), pp. 52-56. Retrieved October 5, 2006, from ProQuest database.

[6] J. Wilmore, H. Knuttgen (2003), "Aerobic Exercise and Endurance Improving Fitness for Health Benefits," *The Physician and Sportsmedicine,* 31(5). 45. Retrieved October 5, 2006, from ProQuest Database.

[7] N. de Vos, N. Singh, D. Ross, T. Stavrinos, et al. (2005), "Optimal Load for Increasing Muscle Power During Explosive Resistance Training in Older Adults," *The Journals of Gerontology,* 60A(5), pp, 638-647. Retrieved October 5, 2006, from ProQuest Database.

[8] WebMD (Nov. 10, 2010), "Resistance (Strength) Training Exercise"; www.webmd.com/a-to-z-guides/resistance-strength-training-exercise-topic-overview. Accessed online April 4, 2012.

[9] Ellen G. White, *The Health Reformer,* July 1, 1872. Ellen G. White is one of the founders of the Seventh-day Adventist Church. Her life and ministry gave strong evidence of the special guidance of the Holy Spirit.

LIQUIDS

[1] U.S. Department of Health and Human Services, National Institute on Aging, "Hyperthermia"; http://www.nia.nih.gov/health/topics/hyperthermia. Accessed online April 4, 2012.

[2] M. G. Hardinge, *A Philosophy of Health* (Loma Linda University School of Public Health, 1980), p. 37.

[3] H. C. Guyton, J. E. Hall, *Textbook of Medical Physiology* (Philadelphia, Penn.: W.B. Saunders Co., 2000), p. 265.

[4] WebMD, "The Basics of Constipation"; http://www.webmd.com/digestive-disorders/digestive-diseases-constipation#causes. Accessed online April 4, 2012.

[5] E. Braunwald, A. S. Fauci, et al., editors. *Harrison's Principles of Internal Medicine* (New York: McGraw Hill) 2011, pp. 1616, 1617.

[6] A. D. Weinberg, K. L. Minaker, "Dehydration,

Evaluation and Management in Older Adults," Council on Scientific Affairs, American Medical Association, *The Journal of the American Medical Association,* Nov. 15, 1995; 274(19): pp. 1552-1556.

[7] United States Department of Agriculture, "Dietary Guidelines for Americans" (2005), "Adequate Nutrients Within Calorie Needs"; http://www.health.gov/dietaryguidelines/dga2005/document/html/chapter2.htm. Accessed May 24, 2007.

[8] Ellen G. White, *The Ministry of Healing* (Mountain View, Calif.: Pacific Press Publishing Association, 1942), p. 237.

ENVIRONMENT

[1] *World Population Prospects: The 2008 revision;* Population Division of the Department of Economics and Social Affairs of the United Nations Secretariat, June 2009.

[2] World Resources Institute, http://earthtrends.wri.org. Accessed online April 20, 2012.

[3] *National Geographic,* "Deforestation—Modern-day Plague"; http://environment.nationalgeographic.com/environment/global-warming/deforestation-overview/. Accessed online April 4, 2012.

[4] S. Peng, et al. "Rice yields decline with higher night temperature from global warming," *Proceedings of the National Academy of Sciences of the United States of America,* July 6, 2004, p. 101.

[5] David B. Lobell and Christopher B. Field, "Global Scale Climate—crop yield relationships and the impact of recent warming," *Environmental and Earth Science,* March 16, 2007.

[6] Henry Leineweber, Resource Recycling, "California sues biodegradable plastic firms"; http://resource-recycling.com/node/2204. Accessed May 3, 2012.

[7] C. J. Moore, S. L. Moore, M. K. Leecaster, and S. B. Weisberg, 2001, "A Comparison of Plastic and Plankton in the North Pacific Central Gyre," *Marine Pollution Bulletin,* vol. 42, no. 12, pp. 1297-1300.

[8] Blacksmith Institutes Technical Advisory Board, (27):9971-5, E-pub June 28, 2004.

[9] Report of the American Lung Association, "The State of the Air," May 2, 2011.

[10] *American Journal of Respiratory and Critical Care Medicine,* October 2000.

[11] H. G. Ainsleigh, "Beneficial effects of sun exposure on cancer mortality," *American Journal of Preventive Medicine,* January 22, 1993(1), pp. 132-140.

[12] E. Braunwald, A. S. Fauci, et al., editors. *Harrison's Principles of Internal Medicine* (New York: McGraw Hill, 2011).

[13] Matthew 5:44; Luke 6:28.

BELIEF

[1] J. S. Levin, H. Y. Vanderpool, "Is frequent religious attendance really conducive to better health? Toward an epidemiology of religion," *Social Science and Medicine,* 1987; 24(7): pp. 589-600.

[2] J. D. Kark, et al. *American Journal of Public Health,* 1996: 86(3); pp. 341-346.

[3] J. S. Levin, L. M. Chatters, R. J. Taylor, "Religious effects on health status and life satisfaction among black Americans," *The Journals of Gerontology, Series B: Psychological Sciences and Social Sciences,* 1995 May;50(3): pp. S154-163.

[4] C. G. Ellison, "A Race, Religious Involvement and Depressive Symptomatology in a South Eastern US Community," *Social Science and Medicine,* 1995:40(11); pp. 1561-1572.

5   V. J. Shoenback, et al. "Social Ties and Mortality in Evans County GA," *American Journal of Epidemiology*, 1986; 123: pp. 577-591.

6   C. G. Ellison, "Religious involvement and subjective well-being," *Journal of Health and Social Behavior*, 1991 Mar;32(1): pp. 80-99.

7   J. W. Dwyer, L. L. Clarke, M. K. Miller, "The effect of religious concentration and affiliation on county cancer mortality rates," *Journal of Health and Social Behavior*, 1990 Jun;31(2): pp. 185-202.

8   H. G. Koenig, *The Healing Power of Healing Faith*, p.72, 1999 Quoting P H Hardestyn and K M Kirby. "Relation Between Family Religious and Drug Use Within Adolescent Peer Groups," *Journal of Social Behavior and Personality* 10:(1) 1995; pp. 42-30.

9   Amoatin and S. J. Bahr, "Religion, Family and Adolescent Drug Use," *Social Perspectives* 29:(1) 1986; pp. 53-76.

10 H. G. Koenig, *The Healing Power of Faith* (Simon & Schuster: April, 1999), p. 177.

11 J. Marks, "A Time Out," *U.S. News & World Report*, Dec. 11, 1995: pp. 85-97.

12 *Journal of Psychology and Theology*, 1991; 19(1): pp. 71-83.

13 L. Dossey, *Healing Words: The Power of Prayer and the Practice of Medicine* (New York: HarperCollins Publisher, 1993) p. 18.

14 *The SDA Bible Commentary*, vol. 4 (Hagerstown, Md., Review and Herald Publishing Association, 1966), p. 203.

REST

*   The details and the chart in this chapter are based on a March 4, 1997, National Transportation Safety Board (NTSB) press release (www.ntsb.gov/news/1997/970304a.htm; accessed June 19, 2012) and a personal interview between the author and a FAA/NTSB investigator.

AIR

1   World Health Organization, "Tackling the global clean air challenge," Press Release September 2011; http://bit.ly/p90Y2g. Accessed April 4, 2012.

2   J. Weuve, et al, "Exposure to particulate air pollution and cognitive decline in older women," *Archives of Internal Medicine*, 2012; 172(3), pp. 219-227.

3   G. A. Wellenius, et al, "Ambient air pollution and the risk of ischemic stroke," *Archives of Internal Medicine*, 2012; 172(3), pp. 229-234.

4   R. Bhatia, "Policy and regulatory action can reduce harms from particulate pollution," *Archives of Internal Medicine*, 2012; 172(3), pp. 227, 228.

5   D. P. Strachan, A. G. Cook, "Parental smoking and lower respiratory illness in infancy and early childhood," *Thorax*, 1997, 52: pp. 905-914.

6   Ibid., pp. 1081-1094.

7   A. K. Hackshaw, et al, "The accumulated evidence on lung cancer and environmental tobacco smoke," *British Medical Journal*, 1997, 315: pp. 980-988.

8   Ellen G. White, *Steps to Christ* (Hagerstown, Md.: Review and Herald Publishing Association, 1956), p. 68.

TEMPERANCE

1   Ellen G. White, *Patriarchs and Prophets* (Nampa, Id.: Pacific Press Publishing Association, 2002), p. 562.

2   World Health Organization, "Global Status Report on Alcohol and Health" (2011); www.who.int/substance_abuse/publications/global_alcohol_report/en. Accessed online April 4, 2012.

3   Ibid.

4   Ibid.

5   Thomas Babor et al. *Alcohol, No Ordinary Commodity*, second edition (New York: Oxford University Press, 2010), p. 70.

6   Richard K. Ries et al. *Principles of Addiction Medicine*, fourth edition (Philadelphia, Penn.: Wolters Kluwer/Lippincott Williams & Wilkins, 2009).

7   European Alcohol Policy Alliance, "Alcohol and cancer—the forgotten link" (May 2011); www.eurocare.org/library/latest_news/alcohol_and_cancer_the_forgotten_link. Accessed April 5, 2012.

8   World Cancer Research Fund International; www.wcrf.org. Accessed April 5, 2012.

9   David Nutt et al. "Drug Harms in the UK: A multi-criteria analysis," *The Lancet*, early online publication, November 1, 2010.

10 Thomas Babor et al. *Alcohol, No Ordinary Commodity*, second edition (New York: Oxford University Press, 2010), p. 1393.

11 Timothy S. Naimi et al. "Cardiovascular Risk Factors and Confounders Among Nondrinking and Moderate-Drinking US Adults," *American Journal of Preventive Medicine*, 2005; 28(4).

12 Kaye Middleton Fillmore et al. "Moderate Alcohol Use and Reduced Mortality Risk: Systematic Error in Prospective Studies," *Addiction Research and Theory*, 1-31, preview article.

13 Boris Hansel et al. *European Journal of Clinical Nutrition*, 64 (June 2010), pp. 561-568.

14 World Health Organization, Fact Sheets, "Tobacco," July 2011; www.who.int/mediacentre/factsheets/fs339/en/index.html. Accessed April 5, 2012. See also Omar Sharey, Michael Eriksen, Hana Ross, Judith MacKay, *The Tobacco Atlas*, third edition, American Cancer Society, 2009.

INTEGRITY

1   George Ludwig, "Leadership 101: Integrity by Example," www.evancarmichael.com/Sales/3443/Leadership-101-Integrity-by-Example.html. Accessed June 12, 2012.

2   Public Health Leadership Society, "Principles of the Ethical Practice of Public Health, 2002; http://phls.org/CMSuploads/Principles-of-the-Ethical-Practice-of-PH-Version-2.2-68496.pdf. Accessed May 3, 2012.

3   *Journal of Substance Abuse*, vol. 9 (Elsevier Inc., 1997) pp. 107-110.

4   Centers for Disease Control, Morbidity and Mortality Weekly Report, June 1, 2001, vol. 50, no. 21; http://www.cdc.gov/mmwr/pdf/wk/mm5021.pdf. Accessed May 3, 2012.

OPTIMISM

1   Elliott McLaughlin, *CNN World*, October 11, 2010, 3:01 PM EST.

2   Harold G. Koenig, Michael E. McCullough, David B. Larson, *Handbook of Religion and Health* (New York: Oxford University Press, 2001), p. 207.

3   *The Oxford Compact English Dictionary* (England: Oxford University Press, 1996), p. 700.

4   Harold G. Koenig, Michael E. McCullough, David B. Larson, ibid.

5   *New Scientist Life*, "Source of 'optimism' found in the brain," October 24, 2007; www.newscientist.com/article/dn12827-source-of-optimism-found-in-the-brain.html. Accessed April 5, 2012.

6   N. Cousins, *Anatomy of an Illness as Perceived by the Patient* (New York: W. W. Norton & Company, Inc., 1979).

7   R. I. M. Dunbar, Rebecca Baron, et al. *Proceedings of the Royal Society B: Biological Sciences*, March 22, 2012, vol. 279, no. 1731, pp. 1161-1167.

8   L. F. Berkman, S. L. Syme, "Social networks, host resistance, and mortality: a nine-year follow-up study of Alameda County residents," *American Journal of Epidemiology*, 1979, Feb; 109(2): pp. 186-204.

9   D. C. McClelland, "Motivational factors in health and disease," *American Psychologist*, 1989, 44(4): pp. 675-683.

10 C. Conversano, A. Rotondo, et al. *Clinical Practice and Epidemiology in Mental Health*, May 14, 2010; 6: pp. 25-29.

11 Harold G. Koenig, Douglas M. Lawson, *Faith in the Future* (West Conshohocken, Pa.: Templeton Press, 2004), p. 159.

NUTRITION

1   USDA "Dietary Guidelines for Americans, 2000"; www.health.gov/dietaryguidelines/dgac/. Accessed June 19, 2012.

2   USDA "Dietary Guidelines for Americans, 2010"; www.choosemyplate.gov/food-groups/fruits.html. Accessed online June 19, 2012.

3   USDA, SuperTracker; www.choosemyplate.gov/SuperTracker/default.aspx. Accessed June 19, 2012.

SOCIAL SUPPORT

1   Julia Neuberger, "Face to faith," *The Guardian*, January 1, 2010; www.guardian.co.uk/commentisfree/belief/2010/jan/02/social-networking-real-world-online. Accessed April 5, 2010.

2   Abraham Maslow, "Maslow's Hierarchy of Needs: The Motivation Theory and Hierarchy of Needs From Abraham Maslow," March 3, 2011, www.maslowshierarchyofneeds.net/maslows-love-and-belonging-needs. Accessed April 12, 2012.

3   S. Cohen, S. L. Syme (eds.), *Social Support and Health* (Orlando, Fla.: Academic Press, 1985).

4   L. F. Berkman, T. Glass, "Social integration, social networks, social support, and health," *Social Epidemiology* (Oxford, Eng.: Oxford University Press, 2000), pp. 137-173. See also L. F. Berkman, L. Syme, "Social networks, host resistance, and mortality: A nine-year follow-up study of Alameda County residents," American Journal of Epidemiology, 1979; 109: pp. 186-204.

5   E. Stice, J. Ragan, P. Randall (2004), "Prospective relations between social support and depression: Differential direction of effects for parent and peer support," *Journal of Abnormal Psychology, 113*, pp.155-159.

6   V. Battistich, A. Horn, "The relationship between students' sense of their school as a community and their involvement in problem behaviors," *American Journal of Public Health*, December 1997; 87(12): 1997-2001.

7   See W. J. Strawbridge et al., "Frequent Attendance at Religious Services and Mortality over 28 Years," *American Journal of Public Health* 87, no. 6 (1997): pp. 957-961. See also H. G. Koenig et al., "Does Religious Attendance Prolong Survival? A Six Year Follow-Up Study of 3,968 Older Adults," *Journal of Gerontology* 54A (1999): M370-377.

8   Rick Nauert, PsychCentral, "Social Support Helps Women Beat Breast Cancer," January 21, 2011, http://psychcentral.com/news/2011/01/21/social-support-helps-women-beat-breast-cancer. Accessed April 13, 2012.

9   Ibid.

10 Ellen G. White, *Testimonies for the Church*, vol. 2 (Mountain View, Calif., Pacific Press Publishing Association, 1948), p. 534.

11 E. Friedmann, S. A. Thomas, "Pet ownership, social support, and one-year survival after acute myocardial infarction in the Cardiac Arrhythmia Suppression Trial (CAST)," *American Journal of Cardiology*, 1995, 76: pp. 1213-1217.

12 William A. Karlin, Elizbeth Brondolo, and Joseph Schwartz, *Psychosomatic Medicine* (2003), 65:167-176.

13 Adapted from "How to Improve Your Social Skills: 8 Tips From the Last 2500 Years," PositivityBlog; http://www.positivityblog.com/index.php/2007/11/15/how-to-improve-your-social-skills-8-tips-from-the-last-2500-years/.

14 Ellen G. White, *Medical Ministry* (Mountain View, Calif.: Pacific Press Publishing Association, 1963), p. 204.

BIBLE VERSIONS

Photography Credits

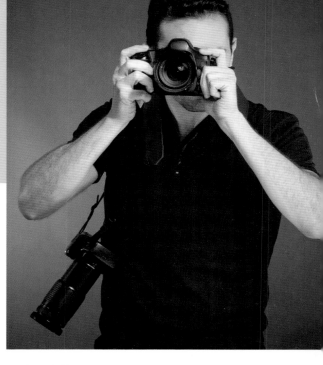